T'ai Chi Ch'uan and I Ching

Da Liu has been teaching and practising T'ai Chi Ch'uan for over fifty years. Born in China, he now lives in the United States and is the author of many books, including *T'ai Chi Ch'uan and Meditation*, *The Tao and Chinese Culture*, *The Tao of Health and Longevity*, *I Ching Coin Prediction* and *I Ching Numerology*. Some of these titles are published by Arkana.

太極拳與易經

T'AI
CHI
CH'UAN
AND
I CHING

Second Edition

Da Liu

ARKANA

ARKANA

Published by the Penguin Group
Penguin Books Ltd, 27 Wrights Lane, London W8 5TZ, England
Viking Penguin, a division of Penguin Books USA Inc.
375 Hudson Street, New York, New York 10014, USA
Penguin Books Australia Ltd, Ringwood, Victoria, Australia
Penguin Books Canada Ltd, 2801 John Street, Markham, Ontario, Canada L3R 1B4
Penguin Books (NZ) Ltd, 182–190 Wairau Road, Auckland 10, New Zealand

Penguin Books Ltd, Registered Offices: Harmondsworth, Middlesex, England

First published in the USA by Harper & Row 1972
First published in Great Britain by Routledge & Kegan Paul 1974
Second edition 1981
Published by ARKANA 1990
3 5 7 9 10 8 6 4 2

Printed and bound in Great Britain by
Cox & Wyman Ltd, Reading, Berks.

FOREWORD

I have been teaching T'ai Chi Ch'uan, a Chinese form of body movement, to students from all parts of the world for more than twenty years. Frequently I am asked questions about the practice of T'ai Chi Ch'uan: "Will it improve my physical condition?" "Can it relieve stress and tension?" "Will it put me 'in tune' with my body?" "In what ways is T'ai Chi Ch'uan related to Chinese thought?"

Many people who know even a little about T'ai Chi Ch'uan realize that it draws upon *yin* and *yang,* the passive and active principles of Chinese philosophy. They also know that the popular contemporary pastime of casting the *I Ching* is based on a world-view that utilizes the same concepts. Quite properly they have asked, "What is the relationship between T'ai Chi Ch'uan and the *I Ching*?" Such a connection exists in that each T'ai Chi movement is related to a particular hexagram of the *I Ching.* This relationship holds vital clues to a deeper understanding of Chinese thought which, like all valid world-views, is based on knowledge of the self gleaned from the practical experience of meditation. The movements of T'ai Chi Ch'uan and the hexagrams upon which they are based are both methods of describing the circulation of psychic energy in the body of the meditator.

This book is, to my knowledge, the first to explain in the English language the connection between the T'ai Chi movements and the hexagrams. I am well aware that in contemporary America the *I Ching* is regarded almost solely as a book of prediction. T'ai Chi Ch'uan is known in America as a physical exercise for relaxation and self-defense. While these views of T'ai Chi and the *I Ching* are not incorrect, they are very much like judging the value of a precious jewel by the opulent case in which it rests. The case may be attractive, arrayed in velvet and gold, but it is nothing in comparison to the jewel buried securely inside.

T'ai Chi Ch'uan and the *I Ching* both allow one to discover that most precious jewel, the nature of the Tao. They do this by revealing the secrets of the Circulation of Light, the circulation of psychic energy in meditation. T'ai Chi Ch'uan and the *I Ching* are the keys by which the theoretical philosophy of Taoism can be converted to a practical way of knowledge. Of course, even this kind of knowledge, if practiced without an experienced master and if practiced under the wrong conditions, is not likely to lead anywhere.

I began my studies in 1928 in Kiang-su in East China under the famous Sun Lu-tang, a master who founded the Sun School of T'ai Chi Ch'uan. Later, I traveled to the Southwest Provinces where I met and studied with great T'ai Chi masters. I then changed from the Sun to the Yang School, the form which I teach today.

I hope that this book will enable the earnest seeker to realize the depth and magic of both the *I Ching* and T'ai Chi Ch'uan. I also hope that it will encourage the T'ai Chi student to greater proficiency and inspiration in his practice.

Many people helped me in the preparation of this book. They have my sincere appreciation: Herbert Cohen, Earl George, Joseph Month, Barbara Rosenthal, Richard Shulman, Carol Southern, Olive Wong, and James Wyckoff.

Da Liu

New York City
December 1971

CONTENTS

FOREWORD   v

PREFACE TO THE SECOND EDITION   xi

I. INTRODUCTION

T'ai Chi Ch'uan Today   1
The Origin of T'ai Chi Ch'uan   3
The *I Ching*   5
Yin-Yang and Taoism   7

II. THE PRINCIPLES OF MOVEMENT IN T'AI CHI CH'UAN

Mind   10
Inner Movement   10
Outer Movement   11
How to Practice   13

III. THE FORMS

PART ONE

FIRST SERIES

1. Beginning of the T'ai Chi Ch'uan   16
2. Grasp Bird's Tail *(left)*   16

SECOND SERIES

3. Push Up   18
4. Pull Back   18
5. Press Forward   18
6. Push Forward   18
7. Single Whip   18

THIRD SERIES

   8. Play Guitar *(right)*   20
   9. Pull Back   20
  10. Step Forward and Strike with Shoulder   20
  11. White Crane Spreads Wings   22

FOURTH SERIES

  12. Brush Knee and Push *(left)*   22
  13. Play Guitar *(left)*   22
  14. Brush Knee and Push *(left)*   25
  15. Step Forward and Punch   25
  16. Draw Back and Push Forward   26
  17. Cross Hands   26

PART TWO

FIRST SERIES

  18. Bring Tiger to the Mountain   27

SECOND SERIES

  19. Fist Under the Elbow   27
  20. Step Back and Repulse Monkey   29
  21. Slant Flying   29

THIRD SERIES

  22. Needle at Sea Bottom   29
  23. Play Arms Like a Fan   31
  24. Turn Body and Strike Fist to Back   31

FOURTH SERIES

  25. Step Forward and Punch   31
  26. Hit Tiger *(left, then right)*   31
  27. Kick with Toes   33
  28. Hit Opponent's Ears with Fists   34

FIFTH SERIES

  29. Turn Body and Kick   34
  30. Brush Knee and Push *(left)*   36
  31. Wave Hands Like a Cloud   36
  32. Single Whip   36

SIXTH SERIES

33. Snake Creeps Down   36
34. Golden Cock on One Leg *(left, then right)*   39
35. High Pat on Horse *(right)*   40
36. Separate Feet and Kick *(right)*   40
37. High Pat on Horse, and Separate Feet and Kick *(left)*   41

SEVENTH SERIES

38. Turn Body and Kick   41
39. Brush Knee and Push *(left, then right)*   42
40. Step Forward and Punch to Opponent's Lower Abdomen   43

EIGHTH SERIES

41. Fair Lady Works at Shuttles *(left, right, left, and right)*   43
42. Grasp Bird's Tail *(left)*   44

NINTH SERIES

43. Snake Creeps Down   44
44. Step Forward, Seven Stars   46
45. Ride Tiger to the Mountain   46
46. Turn Body and Do Lotus Kick   46

TENTH SERIES

47. Shoot Tiger   48
48. Circle Fist   48
49. Step Forward and Punch   50
50. Cross Hands—Conclusion of T'ai Chi Ch'uan   50

IV. THE FORMS AND THE HEXAGRAMS

Beginning of the T'ai Chi Ch'uan: *Chin*   51
Grasp Bird's Tail and Push Up: *Ch'ien*   52
Pull Back: *K'un*   53
Press Forward: *K'an*   53
Push Forward: *Li*   53
Single Whip: *Ko*   54
Play Guitar: *Sui*   54
Step Forward and Strike with Shoulder: *Ta Chuang*   55
White Crane Spreads Wings: *Pi*   56
Brush Knee and Push: *Ku*   56
Step Forward and Punch: *Yu*   57
Cross Hands: *Ming I*   58
Bring Tiger to the Mountain: *Ken*   58

Fist Under the Elbow: *I*   59
Step Back and Repulse Monkey: *Tun*   60
Slant Flying: *Huan*   60
Needle at Sea Bottom: *Hsiao Kuo*   61
Play Arms Like a Fan: *Ta Ch'u*   62
Turn Body and Strike Fist to Back: *Ta Kuo*   62
Hit Tiger: *I*   63
Kick with Toes: *Meng*   64
Hit Opponent's Ears with Fists: *Shih Ho*   64
Turn Body and Kick: *Wu Wang*   65
Wave Hands Like a Cloud: *Chun*   66
Snake Creeps Down: *Shih*   66
Golden Cock on One Leg: *Chung Fu*   67
High Pat on Horse: *Lu*   68
Separate Feet and Kick: *Chen*   68
Step Forward and Punch to Opponent's Lower Abdomen: *Ch'ien*   69
Fair Lady Works at Shuttles: *Chieh*   69
Step Forward, Seven Stars: *Feng*   70
Ride Tiger to the Mountain: *Chien*   71
Turn Body and Do Lotus Kick: *Wei Chi*   71
Shoot Tiger: *Hsieh*   72
Circle Fist: *Ting*   72

V. T'AI CHI CH'UAN USED FOR SELF-DEFENSE

Single Push Hand   74
Double Push Hands   75
Moving Double Push Hands   76
Ta Lu   77

VI. TAOIST MEDITATION AND T'AI CHI CH'UAN   80

VII. THE WAXING AND WANING OF CH'IEN AND K'UN AS APPLIED TO THE PRACTICE OF T'AI CHI CH'UAN   85

NOTES   103

PREFACE TO
SECOND EDITION

The first British edition of my *T'ai Chi Chu'an and I Ching*, published in 1974 has been through many printings. It has been a very successful book and is certainly proof of the growing popularity of T'ai Chi Chu'an in the West in recent years.

Subsequently I wrote another two books about the *I Ching: I Ching Coin Prediction*, published in 1974, which has been translated into German, French, Dutch and Italian; and *I Ching Numerology* which came out in 1979. Thus the West has become steadily more informed about the relation of the *I Ching* to Chinese philosophy as a whole.

A few practitioners of T'ai Chi Chu'an still doubt that it is closely related to the *I Ching*. Even some books on T'ai Chi Chu'an refer to the *I Ching* only in passing, never in detail. To make the link between the *I Ching* and T'ai Chi Chu'an more convincing, a new chapter on the waxing and waning of *Ch'ien* and *K'un* as applied to the practice of T'ai Chi Chu'an has been added. The phrase T'ai Chi itself originally comes from the *I Ching*. It has wide use in Chinese culture, being found in areas as varied as medical science, meditation, and geomancy, as well as in the exercise of T'ai Chi Chu'an. Whatever the discipline to which it is applied, the concept is rooted in the *I Ching*.

I Ching is translated into English as *The Book of Changes*, but actually has three meanings: "ease," "change," and "changelessness." The basic principle of T'ai Chi Chu'an is derived from all three. First is "ease," for the form should be comfortable and easy. Second is "change"; the form constantly changes from *yin* (heavy) to *yang* (light), never stopping. The exercise also involves mutual change. Always the weight shifts from left to right or right to left. Even though there is this unceasing change, the body should still keep its balance and be centered. The mind is always peaceful and relaxed inside. Thus the exercise embodies changelessness.

It is appropriate to mention in this preface the longstanding tradition of cultural exchange between Britain and China, of which this volume is a part. The cultural relations begin in the early nineteenth century when many British missionaries came to China. They studied Chinese and translated Chinese books into English. James Legge (1815–97) was one of the most successful. He came to China in 1840 and left in 1865. In these twenty-five years he translated the *Five Classics of Confucius* and *The Sacred Books of China*, including the *Tao-Te-Ching* of Lao-Tze, and the writings of Chuang-Tzu. These were the first translation of these works in English.

I am happy to be able to add the present work to the literature on this subject.

I am thankful to the following for their help in completing this manuscript: Dr John Lad, Jim Hickey, David Sheinkin, Reggie Jackson, Susan Delone, and Dr Maurice Valency.

I. INTRODUCTION

T'ai Chi Ch'uan Today

Although its roots are in ancient China, T'ai Chi Ch'uan is very suitable for tense Westerners. It has the advantages of regular exercise combined with a definite emphasis on the gracefulness and slowness of pace that Western society so conspicuously lacks. T'ai Chi Ch'uan can give those who live in industrialized fast-paced cities a compensating factor in their lives. It relaxes the mind as well as the body. It helps digestion, quiets the nervous system, benefits the heart and blood circulation, makes joints loose, and refreshes the skin.

Any age group can practice T'ai Chi. Liu Sho-ting, a contemporary T'ai Chi master, at eighty-four years of age still teaches it to students. He began to practice after he had a heart attack at the age of sixty. In three years, he was out of danger with a stronger and more vigorous body than before.

In the beginning one needs a large space to practice. More advanced students need only four square feet. The movements can be performed without any cumbersome equipment. Teamwork, although sometimes enjoyable, is unnecessary. Only for pushing hands, the T'ai Chi form of self-defense, are two people required. Appropriate in any season of the year and in any weather, like the Tao itself, T'ai Chi is unlimited in its benefits and the conditions in which it reveals its nature. It is best to practice the forms two times a day: in the morning when arising and before going to bed in the evening. During lunch, it can be done in the office. Throughout the world T'ai Chi is performed for a variety of reasons. Dance and theater schools in America use it as part of their training routines. Medical institutions in China use it to aid in restoring health. In New York it is even taught in old-age homes. For daily exercise and for maintaining health it is an ideal regimen.

Personally, I agree with the great master Chang San-feng when he said, "This exercise will lead many practitioners to health, happiness, and longevity. The defense is secondary." I don't like to emphasize competition or pushing hands in my classes. Still, in its proper place, T'ai Chi Ch'uan is an effective defense form and I teach it when I am sure sufficient forms have been mastered.

T'ai Chi can help both men and women enhance their personal appearance. Beauty is not confined to the face but penetrates the whole body. The relaxed, gentle movements of T'ai Chi Ch'uan keep the body from being tense and awkward. The forms also keep the body erect and well-postured. Since muscular tension drains the fine blood vessels of the face and hands from an adequate supply of blood, the relief provided by T'ai Chi corrects this condition, pouring color and life into neglected parts as water to a flower. Adequate oxygen and blood circulation prevent a person from appearing old.

There are many schools of T'ai Chi Ch'uan. The Yang School, which I follow, is derived from the Chen School. Four generations have continued the Yang School considerably beyond its predecessor. The Yang School has great influence in Chinese society and is also the most popular there and abroad. Another, the Wu School, was developed out of the Yang School in the 1920s. It is popular mostly in Hong Kong. One more, the Sun School, was created by Sun Lu-tang, a master of symbolical forms. But it is not too popular today. Sun is better known for his work in *Sheng I* and *Pa-Kua* (Eight Trigram) boxing.

The high forms, in which the body is kept upright, are best for the beginner and the old person. The more advanced student should use the low forms with their large steps and low-postured body, necessitating particularly loose joints and flexible limbs. The middle forms, neither high nor low, are suitable for the average student.

The long form of the Yang School has 108 different postures. It is like the Yangtze River, long but gently flowing. It lasts fifteen to twenty minutes when fully comprehended. The professional T'ai Chi student should learn this form. The short form, which is recommended for the average student, is much easier to learn, comprising about fifty forms and taking from seven to ten minutes or less to perform. It is good for the office worker and for people who wish to improve their health and can be practiced two or three times a day.

If you wish to learn T'ai Chi Ch'uan, you must first be positively determined in mind. In order to achieve proficiency daily practice is desirable. It must become an essential part of your life. Second, you should find a good teacher. He will give you a combination of correct forms and the deep philosophy underlying it. He will inspire you to achieve the strong yet subtle concentration necessary to master these forms.

The Origin of T'ai Chi Ch'uan

Before pursuing the shadowy history of T'ai Chi Ch'uan, it is well to note that the hexagrams, the *I Ching,* the concept of *yin-yang,* and the sophisticated methods and philosophy of Taoist meditation preceded it. While the inspiration for T'ai Chi may very well have come from nature—from the observation of animals, for instance— its actual source of energy lies entirely within.

Many credit Chang San-feng of the Sung Dynasty (960–1278) with the development of T'ai Chi Ch'uan in the twelfth century. Others say that he lived in the thirteenth or even in the sixteenth century. He is said to have had two important predecessors, an Indian monk named Ta Mo, who came to China to practice meditation, and a wood-cutter named Hsü Hsuan-ping, who lived a century and a half after Ta Mo (around 750). Ta Mo supposedly invented his *Shiao-lin* exercise, a series of movements similar to some of the T'ai Chi movements, for the physically degenerated monks of the Shiao-lin Monastery. He wished to strengthen their bodies so that they could be a more secure temple for the soul. Hsü Hsuan-ping performed the Long Boxing Exercise, a series of movements which contain many forms of contemporary T'ai Chi, such as Single Whip, White Crane Spreads Wings, and Step Forward, Seven Stars.

But legend has it that the firmest and most complete foundations of the T'ai Chi Ch'uan came from the famous Taoist Chang San-feng, known as the Immortal. He is said to have been an ardent follower of Confucius and to have had a strong interest in the *I Ching*. He had a prominent position as a magistrate in the Chung-san district in China. Later he gave up his official capacities to become a hermit. Still alive in the Ming Dynasty, he continued to study under various enlightened Taoists. Traveling from place to place, he learned techniques of meditation and the martial arts.

According to the legendary story, Chang San-feng, in the house meditating at noon, heard an unusual noise in the courtyard. Looking down from his window, he saw a snake with raised head, hissing in challenge to a crane in the tree above. The crane flew down from the pine tree and attacked the snake with its swordlike beak. But the snake turned its head aside and attacked the crane's neck with its tail. The crane used its right wing to protect its neck. Then the snake darted against the crane's legs. The crane raised its left leg and lowered its left wing to combat the assailant. Stabbing again and again, the bird was unable to make a solid blow. The snake, twisting and bending, was always out of reach. After a while, tired of fighting, the crane flew back to the tree and the snake slithered into the hole in the tree trunk. There they rested in preparation for their encounter the following day.

Chang San-feng watched this performance from his window again and again. From it he realized the value of yielding in the face of strength. In the combat of the crane and the snake, he saw in living form the principle of the *I Ching:* the strong changing to the yielding and the yielding changing to the strong. He remembered the teaching: "What is more yielding than water? Yet back it comes to wear down the stone." The great master studied the crane and the snake, the wild animals, the clouds, the water and the trees bending in the wind. He codified these natural movements into a system of exercise. From the action of the crane came the form White Crane Spreads Wings. From the action of the snake came Snake Creeps Down. The crane attacking with his beak gave Brush Knee and Push. Constructing other forms based on the movements he had seen, he also adapted Shiao-lin martial sets to the idea of Taoist meditation.

Chang San-feng taught his disciples Taoism and meditation in the White Clouded Temple in Peking West Mountain. He created another school for T'ai Chi and other exercises in Hu-pei Province on the Wu-tang Mountain. This was known as the Wu-tang School and stood in contrast to the Shiao-lin School for several hundred years. We owe the present forms of T'ai Chi to numerous masters who utilized and perfected their techniques over many centuries.

The *I Ching*

The *I Ching* is one of the first efforts of the human mind to place itself in the universe. A collection and interpretation of a series of sixty-four 6-line figures called hexagrams, it has exerted a living influence in China for three thousand years. The individual hexagrams predate the *Book of Changes*. They were preserved on wood tablets long before they were recorded by King Wen in 1150 B.C.

The *I Ching* eventually became the most important of the Five Confucian Classics *(History, Odes, Ritual, Spring and Autumn,* and *Change)* and was the only one of these spared when Emperor Ch'in Shih Huang Ti ordered all the ancient books burned in 213 B.C. Its antiquity and worth is substantiated by its use as a common source for both Confucian and Taoist philosophies for many centuries.

The Chinese character for *I* in *I Ching* signifies both change and changelessness. It is constructed from the characters that make up those of the sun and moon, which, although appearing and disappearing each day and night, remain a changeless feature of the heavens. *I* also denotes easiness and clarity. These meanings suggest the clarity with which nature, society, and the individual are revealed through the agency of the sixty-four hexagrams. *Ching* means a book or classic written by a sage.

Each of the hexagrams consists of two 3-lined figures called trigrams. There are eight basic trigrams constructed from a combination of unbroken and broken lines. The trigrams, like the mathematical symbols x and y, can stand for many things. For instance, the trigram *Ch'ien* can mean heaven (the natural world), leader or king (the social realm), father (family relationship), head (part of body), strength (quality), and other things as well. Combined in a hexagram, the symbols acquire a distinct composite meaning. Each line shows a different aspect of the situation pictured by the hexagram.

The creation of the eight trigrams is attributed to Fu Shi, the legendary Chinese sage who reputedly lived during the age of hunting and fishing around 5,000 years ago. By studying and observing heaven, earth, animal tracks, and his own body, he devised the broken and unbroken line as symbols of the fundamental nature of the universe. From these, he constructed eight trigrams, each of which stood for an aspect of nature, society, and the individual.

The origin of the sixty-four hexagrams is unclear. Supposedly, they were created after the time of Fu Shi. King Wen composed his book during his captivity, following his arrest by Emperor Shing Chu. He spent seven years in prison, studying the hexagrams by night and day. He structured his findings in the form of predictions which implied other meanings besides divination. King Wen's codification led to a commentary consisting of the Judgment, the Image, and the text attached to individual lines of the hexagrams. His son, the Duke of Chou, completed the work by adding to the text a commentary known as the Decision, which clarifies the Judgment of the hexagram and discusses the philosophy out of which the prediction develops.

The last contribution to the I Ching was made by the great Chinese philosopher Confucius, who, with his students, wrote a complete and detailed treatise on the philosophy of the book as it then existed. This section is called the Ten Wings. The Ten Wings, which are like a book review, explain and analyze the history, philosophy, and spiritual meaning of the book. They include a detailed discussion of the trigrams (Eighth Wing, or chapter), a commentary on the Images (Third and Fourth Wings), and miscellaneous notes on the hexagrams (Tenth Wing).

Thus, the I Ching through the centuries evolved from simple unbroken and broken lines into a complete philosophical book.

The first English translation of the I Ching was made in the nineteenth century by James Legge, a Scottish missionary and scholar. Since that time, more than twenty English-language editions have been published. The best-known English version of the I Ching was first translated into German earlier in this century by Richard Wilhelm. Rendered into English by Cary F. Baynes, with an introduction by the distinguished psychiatrist Carl G. Jung, this version, from which we shall often cite text, is arranged in three books: Book I consists of the sixty-four hexagrams and the Judgment, Images, and text for each line written by King Wen. Book II contains the Ten Wings written by Confucius, his students, and his disciples. Book III, the most useful in prediction, is made up of the hexagrams with the commentaries of both Confucius and the Duke of Chou. The commentaries discuss the meaning and symbolism of each hexagram.

The *I Ching* also gives practical advice on matters not directly connected with divination or philosophy. It includes information on government, numerology, astrology, cosmology, meditation, and military strategy. John Blofield, in his version of the *I Ching,* says that is was used regularly by generals of the Japanese army during the Russo-Japanese War in 1904–1905. Although its wisdom took root in China, the *I Ching* is an integral part of the cultural heritage of Japan, Korea, Vietnam, and other Far Eastern countries. Its impact on the West is just beginning. At this moment the hexagrams are being developed for computer use, and in this form their wisdom will be available to the uninitiated on an entirely different level.

> The Changes is a book
> From which one may not hold aloof.
> Its tao is forever changing—
> Alteration, movement without rest,
> Flowing through the six empty places;
> Rising and sinking without fixed law,
> Firm and yielding transform each other.
> They cannot be confined within a rule;
> It is only change that is at work here. . . .
>
> They also show care and sorrow and their causes.
> Though you have no teacher,
> Approach them as you would your parents.[1]

Yin-Yang and Taoism

The concept of *yin-yang* is often associated with the name of Lao-tzu. Actually it was discovered and used for something like 4,800 years, several thousand years before Lao-tzu and his famous work, the *Tao Teh Ching,* which enunciated the principles of Taoism. The polarities of *yin* and *yang* exist everywhere, in everything and in every time. In the *I Ching* and Taoist thought heaven is *yang,* earth is *yin;* sun is *yang,* moon is *yin;* man is *yang,* woman is *yin;* firmness is *yang,* yielding is *yin.* In the body, the head is *yang* and the belly is *yin.* Since this duality penetrates all of nature we can, of course, find many other examples.

In T'ai Chi Ch'uan the light foot is *yang* and the heavy, firmly placed foot, *yin*. The light forms are *yang;* the heavy are *yin*. A *yang* form will always follow a *yin* form, one going forward or to one side, the other going back.

Lao-tzu, although not the inventor of this concept, expounded it magnificently. He lived between 604 and 531 B.C., though legend has it that he lived to be several hundred years old. In his youth he was supposedly a librarian who kept documents in the time of the Chu Dynasty. But he gave up his job and went to live alone as a hermit in far West China. He is said to have been the Immortal who passed on to Buddha the secret of immortality. Legend also has it that hè met Confucius and awed him by his superior wisdom. Whatever the validity of these stories, Lao-tzu expounded the philosophy of the Tao most eloquently.

The spirit of Taoism demands a vigorous and wholehearted devotion to Truth and a rather secondary interest in secular affairs if they conflict with devotion. Perhaps this is why many Taoist masters have been accused of laziness and unwillingness to assume responsibilities. One such story illustrating the Taoist attitude toward the world is told about the great master Chuang-tzu, whose writings concerning Taoism are said to be more precise and complete than those of his predecessor, Lao-tzu. He lived around 370 to 300 B.C.

It seems that one day Chuang-tzu was fishing in the Pu River when two civil servants arrived to speak to him. They came with a message from the King of Ch'u: "I wish to trouble you by putting you in charge of everything within my territories."

But Chuang-tzu did not drop his fishing rod. Without looking at the officials, he said, "I hear that in Ch'u there is a sacred tortoise shell whose wearer, the tortoise, died three thousand years ago. And I hear the king who sent you keeps this shell in his ancestral temple in a sacred hamper covered with a sacred cloth. Was it better for the tortoise to die and to leave its shell to be honored? Or would it have been better for that tortoise to live and keep on dragging its tail through the mud?" (In China, tortoises are said to live forever.)

The two officials responded, "Why, it would have been better for it to live and to continue to draw its sacred tail after it over the mud."

"Go your ways," said the sage, matter-of-factly. "I will continue to drag my tail after me through the mud."

Despite this attitude, Taoism did, in fact, intrude its influence into Chinese civil affairs. At the same time the great Taoist master Wang Chen taught, two Taoist strategists, Sun-pin from the state of Chi and Pong-chuen, a general from the state of Wei, became enmeshed in a military struggle against each other. At the end Sun-pin killed Pong-chuen, and Taoism was projected for the first time into a political and military struggle.

Although prayer, rituals, and magical spells have been associated with Taoist practice, as well as traditions of politics and military strategy, the real contribution of Taoism has been to the inner life of man. Its various schools of nonbeing, nonaction, inner and outer elixir have all pointed to the fact that before man can understand the world, he must understand himself. A key part of Taoist practice, therefore, has been the act of meditation. In meditation one learns to focus and direct energies which are usually squandered in the mundane perceptions of the five senses. In Taoist meditation these energies are directed through two main channels: *Tu Mu,* a channel along the spinal column from the base of the spine, where a psychic center called *wei lu* is located, to a psychic center at the top of the head called *ni wan* and over the head to the upper lip; and *Jen Mu,* a channel which passes down the front of the body to the genital region *(huei yin).*

Taoist teaching utilizes both T'ai Chi Ch'uan and the hexagrams to demonstrate the flow of psychic energy *(chi)* along these two channels. The movements of the *chi* are called the Greater and the Lesser Heavenly Circulation. The movements of the arms and legs in T'ai Chi Ch'uan, along with the turns and posturing of the body, help to picture the flow of *chi* during meditation. Also, the very structure of the hexagrams can be used to picture the human body, the two top lines being the head, the middle lines being the chest, and the bottom two being the lower part of the body. The *I Ching* itself can be read as a manual describing the course of the *chi* in meditation and as a guide to the temptations and goals of the meditator.

II. THE PRINCIPLES OF MOVEMENT IN T'AI CHI CH'UAN

The movements of T'ai Chi Ch'uan are based on the coordination of the mind, the inner body, and the outer body.

Mind

It is essential for the mind of the student to be still and concentrated. If the mind is not resolute, the forms will not be achieved. The right mental attitude for practicing is concentrated quietness. This is also the attitude of meditation, in which the outside moves inside. But in T'ai Chi Ch'uan the opposite occurs: the inside moves outside.

Inner Movement

BREATHING

Buddhists refer to breathing as the wheel of law which turns uniformly and unceasingly. Breath is the energy of life. Without breath, there is no life. Taoists regard it as one of the three treasures of the body. The T'ai Chi practitioner regulates his breathing in harmony with the movement of his body to achieve health and the coordination required for self-defense.

Breathing is not only a matter of inhalation and exhalation. It also involves the circulation of the inner vital force called *chi*. When mind, breath, and sexual energy are brought together, *chi* is produced. In order to accomplish deep inner breathing, one must concentrate the *chi* into a psychic center known as the *tan tien,* located three inches below the navel. The *tan tien* may be compared to the boiler of a steam engine. When the mind concentrates there, heat is developed. The excess energy, like the excess water evaporated in the boiler, is then distributed to the rest of the body, propelling the limbs of the T'ai Chi player.

This process of concentration and circulation of *chi,* in turn, produces another substance which we may call spirit, or in Taoist terminology, *shen.* The conversion of one inner essence into another can be likened to an alchemical process. Sexual energy, often referred to literally in the Taoist texts as sperm, is converted into *chi* by mind concentration. Then *chi* is refined to become spirit (or *shen*). The *shen* is further refined to become emptiness *(shu).* In this manner the inner vital force is changed from one state to another, just as the matter of common experience goes through various phases from solid to liquid to gas. According to legend, the master who has reached emptiness has developed an indestructible body and has achieved immortality.

BLOOD CIRCULATION

Like breathing the circulation of the blood is essential to life. The breath controls the circulation of the blood. The T'ai Chi Ch'uan student uses movement to help the *chi,* the inner energy, accelerate the circulation of the blood. Blood circulation and *chi* together propel the limbs in much the same way that gas or steam sets a machine in motion.

Outer Movement

The outer movements of the forms of T'ai Chi Ch'uan are based on principles which are an integral part of the T'ai Chi art.

SMOOTHNESS

Movement should be smooth and even. The student executes all the forms at the same tempo. No movement is sudden or abrupt.

From beginning to end the body moves with the same smooth dynamics.

BALANCE

Each form requires balance. The practitioner leans neither forward nor backward, neither to the right nor to the left. If he loses his balance the player will get into difficulty, feeling uncomfortable and perhaps even falling.

CENTERING

The torso of the body should be erect and in a central position. In the back, from the coccyx to the crown of the head, the body of the student should be a straight line. In the front from the crown of the head to the chest and down to the lower abdomen there should also be a straight line. When the body is erect every bone and inner organ is in its proper position.

In using T'ai Chi for self-defense, the player's body is like a bow and arrow which goes directly to its goal. With practice he learns to achieve this accuracy automatically, without having to look or consciously aim his blows. He can apportion his strength correctly because he himself is centered.

Not only the torso, but the lower body must also be centered. The legs and feet are positioned so that they can pivot freely as well as carry heavy weight without injury. The weight should be placed in the middle of the feet, neither on the toes nor on the heels. In this way the practitioner can support his whole body without fatigue.

RELAXATION

Relaxation of the body and mind is crucial today because of the pace of our industrial cities. The ability to relax is a natural human instinct and, when developed, can aid in the prevention of disease. Both physical and mental relaxation are necessary in order to achieve mastery of the art of T'ai Chi Ch'uan. When the whole body is relaxed, the breath can go directly to the abdomen. The oxygen mixed with the blood can then penetrate into the muscles, just as water penetrates soil. The player should relax his thighs and waist so that he can move freely and without tension. When the legs are relaxed, the body is stable and can move very lightly.

CONTINUITY

In the *Book of Changes* every hexagram develops out of the one before it. Likewise in T'ai Chi Ch'uan, each form follows uninterruptedly and naturally from the previous one. In Chinese thought T'ai Chi Ch'uan is compared to a long river that flows freely and peacefully. It is recorded that Confucius, standing by a river, remarked that everything flows on and on like a river.

COORDINATION

Coordination of body, mind, and breathing is essential. The mind directs the breathing which should parallel the direction of the form. When the form is open or forward, the student inhales. When the form is closed or in retreat, he exhales. This movement of the breath allows the lungs to act as a bellows which pushes the stagnant air out and lets the fresh air in. The arms must be coordinated with the legs and the head with the torso so that none of the parts moves at a faster or slower pace than the others.

How to Practice

The student should let the following points guide him in order to achieve perfection of form:

SLOWNESS

T'ai Chi Ch'uan should be performed slowly and carefully so that the utmost quiet will be achieved. When food is chewed slowly, the taste of it can be fully realized and its digestion can supply more nourishment to the body. In the same way the T'ai Chi player moves slowly through the forms to enhance his concentration, energy, breath control, and patience.

HEAVINESS AND LIGHTNESS

The distribution of weight on the feet is constantly shifted. Sometimes the full weight of the body is on one foot while the other foot is completely light. The same principle is followed in the *I Ching* with regard to the changing lines of the hexagrams. A line with the value nine is completely light, while a six is absolute weight. When a six or a nine is received in divination, it means that the line will change to its opposite (broken to unbroken, unbroken to broken) and a new hexagram will be formed. Sometimes the weight in the T'ai Chi forms is 80 percent on one foot and 20 percent on the other. Sometimes it is 70 percent on one and 30 percent on the other. It is constantly changing. Only at the beginning and at the end is the weight placed equally on both feet.

EFFORTLESSNESS

Because ordinary exercises use strength, the result is often tension and fatigue. T'ai Chi Ch'uan, however, is based on effortlessness. Its movements are free and smooth. All unnecessary exertion is avoided. Less strength is used to produce more strength, as with a lever used to move heavy bodies. Moving smoothly and gracefully, without effort, the student achieves his art as naturally as a child in playing.

III. THE FORMS

T'ai Chi Ch'uan was originally divided into three sections, corresponding to the three primal powers—heaven, earth, and man—into which each hexagram of the *I Ching* is divided. Here, however, I have arranged the T'ai Chi movements in two sections. The first section, containing few forms, is light like heaven. The second section, which has more forms, combines earth and man—the two primal powers that stand under heaven.

The forms in the first section are executed toward the south *(Ch'ien)*, north *(K'un)*, west *(K'an)*, and east *(Li)*. These four trigrams are components of the thirty hexagrams which make up Part I of the *Book of Changes*. The forms in the first section are executed either forward or backward, to the left or to the right.

In the second section there are not only more forms, but they are executed closer to the ground and contain more kicks. From Bring Tiger to the Mountain through Fair Lady Works at Shuttles the forms are executed on the diagonal—toward the northeast *(Chen)*, southwest *(Sun)*, southeast *(Tui)*, and northwest *(K'en)*. These four trigrams are part of the hexagrams which make up Part II of the *Book of Changes*.

In this book I have grouped the movements according to series. The forms in each series are related to each other in meaning. I have found that this arrangement makes it easier for the student to learn and retain each form.

Part One

First Series

1. BEGINNING OF THE T'AI CHI CH'UAN

Stand erect, hands easily at sides, palms back. Heels are together, toes slightly apart (Fig. 1).

Sinking slightly with soft knees, shift weight onto right foot and step with left foot, toes straight forward, to the side so that feet are shoulder-width apart. Shift weight to left, and pivot on right heel to move right toes straight forward. Distribute weight evenly on both feet.

Let arms rise upward to shoulder height in front; draw wrists toward shoulders, fingers slightly straightening (Fig. 2).

Continue the circular movement, gently pressing hands down to sides again. The body rises slightly with the arms and sinks again as arms return to sides.

2. GRASP BIRD'S TAIL *(left)*

The left hand reaches up, palm inward, to hold the bird's neck; the right hand moves down as though smoothing the long plumage of the bird's tail.

Shift weight to left leg; pivoting on right heel, turn to right. Simultaneously the right arm rises, elbow bent, with hand at shoulder height; the left arm rises and crosses body at waist level, palm up. The palms are approximately toward each other (Fig. 3).

Shift weight forward onto right foot and pivot on left toes to turn slightly to the left. Step left with left foot, straight forward and a little left. Simultaneously the weight shifts forward on left foot, the left hand moves up to chin level, palm facing in; the right arm returns to right side, and as the body turns to left the right toes move slightly inward (Fig. 4).

Fig. 1

Fig. 2

Fig. 3

Fig. 4

Second Series

3. PUSH UP

Moving most of weight to left leg, the right foot pivots on toes as the body turns right.

Step with right foot slightly forward and a little right, heel first, toes straight ahead. Moving weight forward to right leg, left toes turn in as the right hand curves up and directly ahead to chin level with palm facing in, and left palm touches right palm (Fig. 5).

4. PULL BACK

Turn both hands over so left palm faces up toward right palm and right palm faces down, at the same time moving hands together diagonally to the right and up.

With weight shifting back to left leg, the hands fall down across body to left, the waist moving slightly left (Fig. 6).

5. PRESS FORWARD

The left forearm circles back, palm forward, and returns, pressing forward past left ear to right palm which simultaneously circles up on left side, palm in (Fig. 7). The palms move to the front of the body, the weight shifts to the right leg and pushes the arms forward.

6. PUSH FORWARD

Separate hands to shoulder width. The weight shifts back to the left leg and draws the arms in toward body at shoulder height. The weight moves forward to right leg and arms move forward (Fig. 8).

7. SINGLE WHIP

In this movement the left hand resembles a single whip.

The weight shifts to left leg, which slightly straightens arms, while the right toes are lifted.

Fig. 5

Fig. 6

Fig. 7

Fig. 8

Pivoting on the right heel, turn body 135 degrees, arms still extended and moving with the body.

Shift weight to right foot and pivot on left toes, turning body to face left. Simultaneously left arm moves across body at waist, palm up; right arm extends to right side of body, fingers pinched, hand at shoulder height. The elbow points to the floor (Fig. 9).

With weight on right leg, pivot on left toes to turn left, facing forward, opening arms to front.

Left foot takes a wide step forward and to the left. The weight moves to the left foot, the left hand turns palm over as it moves up to press forward with fingertips at throat height as the right toes move inward, pivoting on heel (Fig. 10).

Third Series

8. PLAY GUITAR *(right)*

With most of weight on left leg, turn right, pivoting on right toes. Arms remain at same height and open at the sides, palms facing forward. Move right leg left onto its heel, keeping the toes straight forward. Simultaneously the palms and arms close in, the left palm facing the right elbow at a five-inch distance (Fig. 11).

9. PULL BACK

Keeping the weight on left leg, draw the right foot back on its toes and close to the left foot, dropping hands toward and alongside the left leg, palms facing leg (Fig. 12).

10. STEP FORWARD AND STRIKE WITH SHOULDER

Step forward with right foot, toes straight, shifting weight to right foot and press body forward to the right side. Simultaneously the left hand moves across the right to lightly touch right wrist (Fig. 13).

Fig. 9

Fig. 10

Fig. 11

Fig. 12

11. WHITE CRANE SPREADS WINGS

Executing this form the T'ai Chi Ch'uan player resembles a crane standing with one foot delicately raised. The right hand is held in front of the forehead while the left remains at the side, indicating the crane's wings. The left foot is raised lightly, resembling the bird's foot.

With weight on right leg, move left leg in toward the right on toes, foot straight ahead and close to right foot. Simultaneously, the left hand moves to the left side, palm back, and the right hand moves up to the right side of the forehead, palm almost forward (Fig. 14).

Fourth Series

12. BRUSH KNEE AND PUSH *(left)*

Sinking slightly on right knee, turn slightly right as right arm lowers, palm up, and left arm moves up and across body to right side, palm down. Step left foot to the left front (Fig. 15).

The left arm continues around and downward to the left to brush across left knee and return to the left thigh.

The right hand comes down from behind the ear, elbow pointed downward, weight is shifted to the left leg as the right hand pushes forward (Fig. 16).

13. PLAY GUITAR *(left)*

The right foot takes a small step by moving slightly in to the left, and weight shifts to right leg. The left foot moves in toward the right and in front onto its heel, and the arms move in reverse of Play Guitar *(right)*. The left foot and left hand extend farther than the right hand and foot (Fig. 17).

Fig. 13

Fig. 14

Fig. 15

Fig. 16

Fig. 17

14. BRUSH KNEE AND PUSH *(left)*

Circle arms around on right side and brush knee and push forward, as in Form 12, stepping left and forward with left foot and shifting weight to the left leg.

15. STEP FORWARD AND PUNCH

Shifting weight to the right, lower the right hand to groin, palm toward body, as left toes turn slightly outward. The right arm bends at elbow and lifts to chest height, making a fist (Fig. 18). Step onto left leg with toes straight ahead as left arm moves across waist level. As weight moves forward onto left leg, right-fisted arm moves forward, pushing through straight ahead (Fig. 19).

Fig. 18

Fig. 19

16. DRAW BACK AND PUSH FORWARD

The left hand moves under right elbow and then pushes outward with back of hand. The right arm curves to the left and back as the fist opens.

Shifting the weight to the right leg, hands are drawn back (Fig. 20). Press forward, arms separating at shoulder height and width, palms down, as weight shifts to left leg.

17. CROSS HANDS

Shift weight to right foot, turn left toes inward, and open hands wide over head. Continue the arms down and forward and then up to cross at the wrists, chest level, palms in. The right foot pivots on toes and steps back to original straight-forward position (Fig. 21). To conclude Part One, repeat Form 1.

Fig. 20   Fig. 21

Part Two

First Series

18. Bring Tiger to the Mountain

Executing this form the player seems to hold the tiger as he steps forward. Tigers are popularly used in T'ai Chi forms owing to the legends of the friendly relationship between the gentle Taoist hermits and the animals of the forest. The tiger, when tamed, could be ridden on mountainous terrain as well as on the flatlands. It could even leap from cliff to cliff, with the masterful Taoist saint riding aloft with perfect tranquillity.

Shift weight to the left leg, make three-quarter turn diagonally to the right and step with right foot. Simultaneously the right arm drops, brushes across right knee with palm facing knee, the palm turning upward on the right side of the knee. The left arm drops back and curves upward to pass the ear as the fingertips press forward and seem to form a ball with right hand. As the arms move the weight shifts to the right, the left foot pivoting on heel (Fig. 22).

After completing Bring Tiger to the Mountain, repeat Forms 4, 5, 6, and 7, performing them on the diagonal rather than straight forward or to the side.

Second Series

19. Fist Under the Elbow

Shift weight to the right leg. The left foot steps left and forward as left arm swings to left, the palm down. The right foot takes a half-step forward and the right arm swings forward with it, the left arm curving down to the side. Putting weight on right leg, the left heel is brought forward to face straight ahead with the left arm moving with it,

Fig. 22

Fig. 23

Fig. 24

Fig. 25

bending at the elbow; the right hand forms a fist which moves under the elbow (Fig. 23).

20. STEP BACK AND REPULSE MONKEY

The left hand grabs the monkey's hand as the right hand pushes the monkey's head away. At the same time, the player steps back.

From preceding form drop right arm to side. Turn left palm to face down and press fingertips forward.

As the body turns to the right, the right arm circles back, and both palms turn up (Fig. 24).

As the body turns forward, the right arm circles around and moves forward past the ear, the left arm falls to the side with the left foot stepping straight back. The right arm moves in front, fingertips pressing forward; the right toes straighten (Fig. 25). The left arm continues back as the body turns to the left.

Repeat these actions on the left side, and then again to the right.

21. SLANT FLYING

The hands sweep upward and downward in a diagonal motion, resembling the flying pattern of a bird winging low over the banks of a river.

Drop right hand across to left thigh (Fig. 26), cross left arm over the right hand. With the right foot take a large step to right and forward on the diagonal (135-degree angle), turning with the body.

The right arm moves diagonally up across the front of the body, palm slanting up. Simultaneously the left toes turn in and the left hand drops to the side (Fig. 27).

After completing Slant Flying, repeat Forms 8, 9, 10, 11, and 12.

Third Series

22. NEEDLE AT SEA BOTTOM

The player brings his hands downward to the sea of breath, the area below the navel. His right hand is held naturally straight, resem-

Fig. 26

Fig. 27

Fig. 28

Fig. 29

bling a needle, as he lowers both hands to knee height—to the bottom of the sea.

Take a small adjustment step to the left with right foot and shift weight to the right, placing left foot on its toes about eight inches in front of right foot. Lower and relax body and let palms drop down to knees, placing the left hand over the right wrist (Fig. 28).

23. PLAY ARMS LIKE A FAN

The hands are spread apart like the two sides of a Chinese folding fan.

Lift body, step forward and to the side with the left foot. Bring the right arm up, palm diagonally sideways to the right. The left arm moves in a forward arc, while the body turns slightly right simultaneously with these arm movements (Fig. 29).

24. TURN BODY AND STRIKE FIST TO BACK

Shift weight to the right and pivot on left heel to turn right. Simultaneously the right forearm moves straight out to the side and makes a fist, while the left arm drops to the side (Fig. 30).

Fourth Series

25. STEP FORWARD AND PUNCH

Turn right toes outward, step forward with left foot, and punch with right fist (Fig. 31). Then shift weight to right, step back with left foot, and pull hands back to left side.

26. HIT TIGER *(left, then right)*

One hand hits the tiger's forehead; another hits his chest.

The left palm turns up, and the right arm circles out, up and over, palm down. The arms then move diagonally across body to left as the left foot steps back (Fig. 32).

The arms continue to circle up and around in front to the right with

Fig. 30

Fig. 31

Fig. 32

Fig. 33

the right toes pivoting out. Shifting weight to the right, as arms continue to circle, step forward with the left foot; the arms move inward, making fists, to either side of the central body line, 11:30 o'clock with the left fist and 5:30 o'clock with the right fist, knuckles forward (Fig. 33).

Repeat the circular arm movements in reverse and continue as before but this time to the right.

27. Kick with Toes

The arms continue to circle up centrally, then out to the sides with palms forward. Here the right leg is lifted, and the toes kick forward and upward (Fig. 34).

The foot relaxes back in lifted position. Both hands move inward, form fists (Fig. 35), and brush down on either side of bent knee.

Fig. 34   Fig. 35

28. Hit Opponent's Ears with Fists

Step forward with right foot, moving weight onto right leg. The arms continue down, out, up, and around toward center to hit the imagined opponent's two ears (Fig. 36).

Fifth Series

29. Turn Body and Kick

Shift weight to the left leg, pivot on right heel to turn toes to the left; simultaneously drop hands (fists released) in an outward arc that circles up to come to rest at chest level, wrists crossed (Fig. 37).

Turn the right toes inward. Turn body to the left side and kick with left foot; the right hand moves up to protect the right temple with palm slightly forward, the left palm is forward and slightly down in the front (Fig. 38).

Fig. 36   Fig. 37

Fig. 38

30. BRUSH KNEE AND PUSH *(left)*

Repeat the movement described for Form 12.

31. WAVE HANDS LIKE A CLOUD

The circular movements of the hands resemble the flowing motions of a cloud passing by in the sky.

With weight on left leg, pivot on right heel and turn to right. Shift weight to right leg and pivot on left heel to continue turn. Simultaneously the left hand moves across the front of the lower trunk, palm up, and the right hand is drawn back with the body in turning (Fig. 39). Left foot then steps forward, in line with and parallel to right foot. The width between the feet is slightly broader than shoulder width.

The body turns left from the waist as the weight moves to the left. Simultaneously the arms exchange: the right arm moves down across the lower trunk, palm up, and the left arm moves up and across to the left as the body turns (Fig. 40).

Alternating from right to left, this movement is repeated seven times.

32. SINGLE WHIP

Repeat the movement described for Form 7.

Sixth Series

33. SNAKE CREEPS DOWN

The hand moves down to the foot as the whole body sinks near to the ground. The motion is flowing and serpentine.

Pivot on right heel and turn right toes to the right side. Shift weight to right leg.

Pivot on left heel to turn toes inward while lowering body to sit almost on right heel. The right arm remains in Single Whip position but straightens. The left arm moves down along the inside of the lower thigh continuing down to pass the calf (Fig. 41).

Fig. 39

Fig. 40

Fig. 41

Fig. 42

Fig. 43

34. GOLDEN COCK ON ONE LEG *(left, then right)*

One hand is held down, the other held up. At the same time, the pose is frozen with one leg held up like a standing cock.

As the left arm continues to move forward across left calf, beginning upward sweep, the left toes turn forward again and the weight shifts to the left leg. The body lifts, the left hand moving up to strike, the right heel pivoting as the toes turn inward. The right arm lowers to the right side (Fig. 42).

The right arm and leg move together as the right arm moves up in an acute angle, palm to the side, and the right knee rises to strike forward, forming a right angle. Simultaneously the left arm drops to the left side (Fig. 43).

Repeat the movement, this time standing on right leg. Arms exchange movements and the left arm and knee move up together (Fig. 44).

Fig. 44   Fig. 45

35. High Pat on Horse *(right)*

In this form the right hand sweeps upward to pat the horse's back as the left hand holds the reins.

Step back onto left foot, lowering left arm to waist level, palm up. The right hand moves up, palm down, across the left palm, as the weight begins to shift forward. As the weight moves forward onto the right leg, the body and hands move diagonally to the right, the hands also moving upward (right hand at forehead height; left hand above waist height) (Fig. 45).

36. Separate Feet and Kick *(right)*

As the weight shifts back onto left leg, the hands drop back and down to the left. Then left arm moves around the left side and to the front of the face, palm open, as right arm moves up to cross wrist with the left arm, palm open. As palms cross, the right foot moves onto its toes (Fig. 46).

The right toes kick low to the right diagonal while the arms slide

Fig. 46   Fig. 47

sideways, left hand at temple with palm forward, and right forearm moving from elbow to the right (Fig. 47).

37. HIGH PAT ON HORSE, AND SEPARATE FEET AND KICK *(left)*

Reverse the movements of Forms 35 and 36 by first stepping back on right leg and dropping right arm to waist height, palm up, and continuing movements on the left side (Fig. 48).

Then the left toes kick low to the left diagonal while the arms slide sideways, right hand at forehead height with palm out, and left forearm moving from elbow to the left (Fig. 49).

Seventh Series

38. TURN BODY AND KICK

Bringing left heel to upper inner right calf, move left arm across body to right, below waist with palm toward body; move the right

Fig. 48   Fig. 49

arm out and down in a low diagonal, and back slightly, body following (Fig. 50).

The right arm propels the body to the left and around in a sweeping
half turn, pivoting on right heel.

Kick forward with left heel while right arm moves up to protect
right temple and left arm strikes forward, palm open (Fig. 51).

39. BRUSH KNEE AND PUSH *(left, then right)*

Step forward and wide with left foot, heel first, toes forward.
Simultaneously brush left hand across left knee and press forward
with right fingers, as before.

Shift weight backward to right leg, brush right knee with right hand,
turn left toes slightly outward, and shift weight to left foot. Step with
right foot, heel first, toes forward, moving weight forward. With this
step the left arm circles back and around and moves past left ear to
press forward with fingertips, the right hand brushing across the right
knee again (Fig. 52).

Fig. 50   Fig. 51

40. STEP FORWARD AND PUNCH TO OPPONENT'S LOWER ABDOMEN

Weight shifts back to left leg, left arm lowers to side and right toes turn slightly outward. Step forward onto left leg, toes forward; brush left knee with left hand; punch forward with right fist to lower part of opponent's abdomen (Fig. 53).

After completing this form, repeat Forms 3, 4, 5, 6, and 7.

Eighth Series

41. FAIR LADY WORKS AT SHUTTLES *(left, right, left, and right)*

As the T'ai Chi player executes this form the hands move from left to right like the back-and-forth movement of a shuttle.

Fig. 52   Fig. 53

Shift weight to right leg and pivot on left heel as far right as possible while left arm moves across body at waist, palm up. Shift weight to left leg, continue movement to northeast corner by pivoting on right toes; the right arm moves slightly down toward left arm. Step with right foot (to northeast), then with left foot.

As weight shifts to left leg, left arm moves up to forehead, palm down, and fingertips of right hand press straight ahead to the left corner (Fig. 54).

Shift weight to right leg, pivot on left heel and turn right as far as possible while left arm moves slightly down to chin as before.

Shift weight to left foot, continuing movement to right by pivoting on right toes. Step with right foot to the right, making a three-quarter turn to the northwest corner. Lift right hand to forehead as before and press left fingertips forward while shifting weight onto right leg (Fig. 55).

Shift weight to left leg, step with right foot to southwest corner, right arm moving down toward waist.

Step in the same direction with left foot and press forward with right fingertips as left arm moves up to protect head, weight moving onto left foot. Right palm pushes through to the southwest corner (Fig. 56).

Shift weight to right leg, pivot on left heel to turn right, and slightly lower left arm. Shift weight to left leg and continue circling to right by pivoting on right toes.

Step right foot far around to complete three-quarter turn and face southeast corner, the right arm lifted to forehead and the left arm pressing forward, left toes turning inward (Fig. 57).

42. GRASP BIRD'S TAIL *(left)*

Repeat the movement described for Form 2; then repeat Forms 3, 4, 5, 6, and 7.

Ninth Series

43. SNAKE CREEPS DOWN

Repeat the movement described for Form 33.

Fig. 54

Fig. 55

Fig. 56

Fig. 57

44. STEP FORWARD, SEVEN STARS

In this form the hands are crossed at the wrists, resembling the seven-star constellation near the pole star.

As the body lifts, turn the right toes in and center the weight on left leg. Move the arms in front to upper chest height and form fists (with back of hands forward) that cross at the wrists, left wrist on inside of the right wrist. Simultaneously move the right foot on its toes in front of left heel (Fig. 58).

45. RIDE TIGER TO THE MOUNTAIN

As he executes this movement the player seems to be riding on a tiger.

Step back on right leg, move weight onto it, and drop left arm to left side. Circle the right hand out to side and up to forehead, palm a little down and forward. As arms move, bring left foot onto its toes in front of right heel (Fig. 59).

46. TURN BODY AND DO LOTUS KICK

A round flower with round leaves, the lotus seems to revolve when the wind blows. In this form the kick is delivered in a circular movement, reminding one of the revolving lotus leaves.

The left leg lifts off the ground slightly forward, and the body turns right to make a 360-degree turn on the ball of the right foot, the arms and legs giving the impetus to the movement (Fig. 60).

Drop right arm diagonally across body to left as far as it will naturally go, palm facing back. Simultaneously turn the left hand to face forward, moving the left arm forward slightly and circling out and back on the left diagonal.

Finish the turn with weight moved entirely onto left leg, knee bending deeply. Simultaneously move arms in front at chest height, palms down.

Lift right leg and touch toes to both palms, arms not moving (Fig. 61).

Fig. 58

Fig. 59

Fig. 60

Fig. 61

Tenth Series

47. SHOOT TIGER

The two hands are held like a bow, the right hand above and the left below. The body and arms move from back to front, imitating the motion of an arrow.

Step forward on right leg and form fists with both hands, knuckles up, the left arm lowering slightly. Punch forward with both fists as the body moves forward (Fig. 62).

48. CIRCLE FIST

Move weight back to left leg and drop arms to sides. Left arm stops at left side and right arm, making a fist, continues clockwise to hit the imagined opponent's head (Fig. 63).

Fig. 62   Fig. 63

Fig. 64

49. STEP FORWARD AND PUNCH

Put weight onto right leg, move left arm across body at chest level above the punching fist, and step forward with left foot. Then punch forward with right fist (Fig. 64).

50. CROSS HANDS—CONCLUSION OF T'AI CHI CH'UAN

Repeat the movement described for Form 17. Then, to conclude T'ai Chi Ch'uan, repeat Form 1.

IV. THE FORMS AND THE HEXAGRAMS

Beginning of the T'ai Chi Ch'uan

CHIN

The opening movement of T'ai Chi Ch'uan is derived from Hexagram 35, *Chin*, which represents Progress. This hexagram is composed of the upper trigram, *Li*, or sun, and the lower trigram, *K'un*, or earth: these elements together symbolize the sun rising above the earth. At the start of the day, the sun moves slowly higher and higher over the earth. This aspect of the sun's movement is captured in the first form.

The student stands erect as he begins the T'ai Chi Ch'uan. His legs are parallel to one another, the stance that is indicated by the lower nuclear trigram *Ken*, or legs (also, arms). His hands then rise slowly from his thighs in a parallel movement. This, too, is suggested by the trigram *Li*, with its two unbroken lines enclosing a broken line. The structure of this trigram calls to mind the epithet, "Strong outside, empty inside," a provocative description of the spiritually advanced man. The student's hands rise from his belly (the lower trigram, *K'un*, also means belly) to his shoulders and down again, slowly and gently.

In the Commentary on the Decision, a section of the *I Ching* in which the hexagrams are interpreted, the following comment is recorded: "Devoted, and clinging to this great clarity, the weak (or, gentle person) progresses and goes upward." This account of the *Chin* movement is further enhanced by the statement given as the Image of the hexagram:

> The sun rises over the earth:
> The image of Progress.
> Thus the superior man himself
> Brightens his bright virtue.

With this, the appropriateness of T'ai Chi Ch'uan is given yet another dimension: not only is it for health and self-defense, it is equally for the development of virtue.[1]

CH'IEN

Grasp Bird's Tail and Push Up

These forms originate with the first hexagram, *Ch'ien,* the Creative. The left palm is held at chin level as though grasping the head of the bird (or dragon). The right hand, placed to the side of the hip as though smoothing the bird's tail, then is raised to the bird's head. The *Book of Changes* says:

> Nine in the second place means:
> Dragon appearing in the field.

The number 9 indicates the unbroken line that is second from the bottom in the hexagram. The phrase "the second place" also refers to the abdomen. The line, "Dragon appearing in the field," is a concrete expression of the first statement, with the dragon represented by the hand and the field understood to be the abdomen.

As the hand, or dragon, flies upward to a place in front of the player's chin, the *Book of Changes* says:

> Nine in the fifth place means:
> Flying dragon in the heavens.

If the hand, however, rises too high and goes above the chin, we can speak of the hand as an arrogant dragon, and the movement becomes stiff and ungraceful.

Nine at the top means:
Arrogant dragon will have cause to repent.

Thus, Push Up reaches its end at the chin, or fifth place, and from there the new form begins.[2]

Pull Back

K'UN

The trigram *K'un,* the Receptive, characterizes Pull Back. The player's hands move downward from his upper right side toward his lower left. The opening words of the Great Commentary of the *I Ching* are appropriate: "Heaven is high, the earth is low."[3]

Press Forward

K'AN

This movement, related to the trigram *K'an,* finds the left hand placed on the right wrist, both hands positioned close to the chest. The hands then press forward, representing the new moon waxing to the full. But in the flow of nature, when the moon is full it begins to wane. The player then separates his hands and rests backward, indicating the waning moon.

Push Forward

LI

Based on the trigram *Li,* this form begins with the hands parallel to each other and in front of the body, a symbol of strength outside and emptiness within. The act of pushing forward recalls the arc of the sun as it goes forward across the heavens.

Push Up, Pull Back, Press Forward, and Push Forward also symbolize the four seasons. When these movements are completed, a new year begins with the transition to the Single Whip.

KO

Single Whip

The Single Whip comes from Hexagram 49, *Ko,* which means Revolution. According to the Commentary on the Decision, "Heaven and earth bring about revolution, and the four seasons complete themselves thereby." The nuclear trigrams *Ch'ien* (which means turning) and *Sun* (which means gentle and wind) suggest the essence of the movement: the body turning with hands still parallel almost 120 degrees from the termination of Push Forward, the previous movement. *Ch'ien* and *Sun* combined give the picture of the body rotating in a gentle flowing motion like a light wind.[4]

SUI

Play Guitar

Sui, Hexagram 17, which denotes Following, is related to Play Guitar *(right).* The upper trigram, *Tui,* may mean joyous or oval-shaped. The lower trigram, *Chen,* sometimes has the meanings of arousing or foot. The upper nuclear trigram, *Sun,* can denote wood or string. The lower nuclear trigram, *Ken,* signifies at times legs, arms, hands, or fingers.

By combining the various elements of the hexagram, we discover a picture of Play Guitar *(right). Tui* suggests a joyous activity, such as playing an instrument. The nuclear trigram *Sun* suggests the pi'pa, an ancient Chinese stringed instrument strummed like a guitar and constructed chiefly from wood. *Ken* indicates the fingers of the guitar-player.

Tui, insofar as it suggests the oval shape, signifies the hands of the combatant as he moves into a strong position, vigorously twisting the opponent's arm. The lower trigram, *Chen,* suggests a firm stance. The foot is aroused, lightly touching the floor and ready to kick.

The T'ai Chi player uses two hands to twist his opponent's arm, as the second line says:

> If one clings to the little boy,
> One loses the strong man.[5]

Step Forward and Strike with Shoulder

TA CHUANG

Step Forward and Strike with Shoulder is taken from Hexagram 34, *Ta Chuang,* which symbolizes the Power of the Great. The primary trigrams are *Chen,* which means arousing or thunder, and *Ch'ien,* which means strong, moving, or forward. The lower nuclear trigram is also *Ch'ien.* The upper is *Tui.* The four strong unbroken lines predominate within and at the lower part of the hexagram. The motion of Step Forward and Strike with Shoulder suggests a goat butting a fence or some like object. Thus the lines in the *I Ching* evoking the goat also evoke this form. In addition, *Tui,* the upper nuclear trigram, denotes goat as one of its multiple meanings. As the third line says:

> The inferior man works through power.
> The superior man does not act thus. . . .
> A goat butts against a hedge
> And gets its horns entangled.

To use Step Forward and Strike with Shoulder as a self-defense technique requires delicacy of aim. If the combatant's body is wrongly placed, the movement will be ineffective. As the Image states:

> Thus the superior man does not tread upon paths
> That do not accord with established order.[6]

PI

White Crane Spreads Wings

The T'ai Chi Ch'uan form White Crane Spreads Wings is based on Hexagram 22, *Pi,* which signifies Grace—beauty of form. The upper trigram, *Ken,* denotes hand or wing. The lower, *Li,* can mean bird or eye. In this form the hands become the crane's wings and one of them is placed above the eyes.

The upper nuclear trigram, *Chen,* suggests movement, feet or forest. When all of its lines are changed, *Chen* becomes *Sun.* Combining *Sun* with *Li,* we have the image of a white bird. The lower nuclear trigram, *K'an,* evokes the image of water. Thus, the hexagram gives the picture of a wild water bird on the outskirts of a forest, the white bird of this T'ai Chi movement.

The fourth line of Hexagram 22 mentions a white horse which comes as if on wings. But the hexagram itself suggests a flying bird, not a horse. The flying creature of the hexagram, with one wing *(Ken)* high and one low, resembles the actual posture of White Crane Spreads Wings.

KU

Brush Knee and Push

Ku, Hexagram 18, is related to Brush Knee and Push. The hexagram signifies Decay. More specifically *Ku* means to work on what has spoiled to remove the source of decay. *Ken,* the upper trigram, signifies hand, leg, or mountain. The lower trigram, *Sun,* means wind, gentle, or willow tree. The upper nuclear trigram is *Chen,* suggesting movement; the lower nuclear trigram is *Tui.* The combined images of the trigrams picture a man stepping forward and pushing. The Image which the *I Ching* gives for *Ku* states: "The wind blows low on the mountain," another way of suggesting Brush Knee and Push.[7] The mountain, of course, is derived from *Ken.* The lower trigram, *Sun,* governs the manner of the form: it is executed gently, like the wind blowing against a willow tree.

Brush Knee and Push is used in self-defense as a block against the kick or hand-blow of the opponent. As he blocks, the combatant points the fingers of his right hand at his opponent's throat.

YU

Step Forward and Punch

Step Forward and Punch comes from Hexagram 16, *Yu,* which denotes Enthusiasm. The upper trigram is *Chen,* meaning thunder, movement, and strength. The lower trigram, *K'un,* means earth or belly. The fourth line, the strong line, is like a fist placed at waist level. The upper nuclear trigram is *K'an,* meaning water or heart. It is appropriate to this movement in which the player punches out at the opponent's heart. The lower nuclear trigram, *Ken,* represents legs and arms, as well as mountain. The leg in Step Forward and Punch must stand firm like a mountain.

Chen often means foot. In relation to this T'ai Chi movement it signifies stepping forward, which is accomplished in a flowing motion, like running water. *K'an* means bow. The solid *yang* line is like an arrow, signifying the punch shot out like an arrow from a drawn bow.

In performing T'ai Chi Ch'uan this whole movement flows like *K'an,* water, and is soft like *K'un,* soil or earth. When Step Forward and Punch is used in an attack, however, it is quick like an arrow and powerful like thunder. Of course, an offensive movement such as this is used only when an attack was previously initiated by an opponent. Like all the techniques of T'ai Chi Ch'uan, this movement is not meant to be used aggressively but can be employed in self-defense.

Cross Hands

The Darkening of the Light, the theme of Hexagram 36, *Ming I,* is also the theme of Cross Hands. The upper trigram of the hexagram is *K'un,* the receptive, earth. The lower trigram, *Li,* means fire as well as light and signifies the sun sinking down beneath the earth. The upper nuclear trigram is *Chen,* which signifies movement or thunder. The three broken lines in the upper trigram mean that the two hands are separate as the movement begins. *Li,* with its broken line between the two unbroken ones, symbolizes the crossed hands, the position that is the goal of this movement. As the *Book of Changes* says:

> Six at the top means:
> Not light but darkness.
> First he climbed up to heaven,
> Then he plunged into the depths of the earth.

The hands rise and then come down to cross, at the end of the movement, before the chest.

The Beginning of the T'ai Chi Ch'uan is derived from the preceding hexagram, *Chin,* the sun rising from the earth. In contrast Cross Hands, which marks the end of the first section, is derived from *Ming I,* which signifies the sun sinking down over the earth.

As the Image puts it:

> Thus does the superior man live with the great mass:
> He veils his light, yet still shines.[8]

Bring Tiger to the Mountain

The *I Ching* Hexagram 52, *Ken,* which means Keeping Still, Mountain, is related to Bring Tiger to the Mountain. The upper and lower trigrams are both *Ken* and can signify arm or hand. The upper nuclear trigram, *Chen,* means embracing. The trigram *Ken* also signifies tiger and mountain. Thus, the hexagram gives the image of a tiger embraced and related in some way to a mountain. The lower nuclear trigram is *K'an,* water. As he performs this movement, the T'ai Chi player seems to throw the tiger and then to let it go back to the mountain. Otherwise he will be in danger. The Commentary on the Decision says:

> When it is time to stop, then stop.
> When it is time to advance, then advance.
> Thus movement and rest do not miss the right time.

Bring Tiger to the Mountain is the beginning of the second section of T'ai Chi Ch'uan. Sometimes the player stops before this form. When he feels ready to advance, he advances. The experienced student rests or continues at the right time.

> Mountains standing close together:
> The image of Keeping Still.
> Thus the superior man
> Does not permit his thoughts
> To go beyond his situation.[9]

Fist Under the Elbow

Fist Under the Elbow is derived from Hexagram 27, *I,* which denotes the Corners of the Mouth (Providing Nourishment). The hexagram is constructed from *Ken,* the upper trigram, which means hand or fingers and *Chen,* which indicates the feet, movement or arousing. Both nuclear trigrams are *K'un,* signifying belly, body, or hidden. In this form one foot is lightly placed with heel on the ground as suggested by the lower trigram, *Chen,* a foot ready for instantaneous arousal, to kick whenever necessary.

In the Fourth Line we read: "Spying about with sharp eyes, like a tiger with insatiable craving."[10] These words suggest the spirit of the form which involves a scrupulous attention to the movements of the opponent as the combatant waits for an opening to strike a sudden blow with the fist or foot or open palm. These blows could be delivered simultaneously by a perfected T'ai Chi master.

Step Back and Repulse Monkey

TUN

Retreat, the essence of Hexagram 33, *Tun,* is also the essence of Step Back and Repulse Monkey. The upper trigram, *Ch'ien,* denotes movement. The lower trigram, *Ken,* means monkey, back, stop, and mountain. Combining the two trigrams, we find move or step back as one of the hexagram's possible meanings. Stop, or repulse, is also suggested by *Ken,* as well as monkey. This combination gives the whole form, Step Back and Repulse Monkey. The upper nuclear trigram, *Ch'ien,* means energy. The lower nuclear trigram, *Sun,* means gentle. Together they imply the gentle application of energy. As the Image says:

> Mountain under heaven: the image of Retreat . . .
> Not angrily but with reserve.

The Commentary on the Decision interprets further: " 'Retreat. Success': this means that success lies in retreating." The implications of this motif are drawn out in Book III of the *I Ching.*

The secret of the T'ai Chi Ch'uan lies in its refusal to use strength against strength. "Retreat and then wait for the right time to counter-attack" is the essence of self-defense according to T'ai Chi.[11]

Slant Flying

HUAN

Huan, Hexagram 59, which means Dissolution, is related to Slant Flying. The upper trigram, *Sun,* connotes wind, penetration, or gentleness. The lower trigram, *K'an,* implies water, ear, or bow. The upper nuclear trigram is *Ken,* meaning leg, hand, or temple (of the head). The lower nuclear trigram is *Chen,* which means foot or movement. Taking the meanings movement (from *Chen*) and leg (from *Ken*), we have a forward step. The hand, as suggested by *Ken,* moves *(Chen)* to strike the opponent's ear *(K'an)* or temple *(Ken).*

Another interpretation is derived from an alternative meaning of the trigram *Sun:* chicken. Again, *K'an* denotes water or river. A chicken, flying slantingly to the sloping banks of a river, will fly low and must continue its trajectory until it finds flat ground or it will drown.

HSIAO KUO

Needle at Sea Bottom

Needle at Sea Bottom is taken from Hexagram 62, *Hsiao Kuo,* which means Preponderance of the Small. Taking the double broken and unbroken line couples as one unbroken line between two broken lines, we get *Big K'an,* which indicates a body of water. Waves piled up upon one another are signified by the double broken lines at the top of *Hsiao Kuo.* The broken lines below signify unfathomable depths. Together these elements give a picture of the sea.

The lower nuclear trigram, *Sun,* implies long, straight, or thread. The upper nuclear trigram, *Tui,* means metal and suggests a needle. Combining these two impressions, we have the form Needle at Sea Bottom.

The upper trigram of *Hsiao Kuo* is *Chen,* meaning movement, arousing, or foot. The lower, *Ken,* means leg or still. The nuclear hexagram is *Ta Kuo* (No. 28), meaning Preponderance of the Great. According to the Image of this hexagram, "The lake rises above the trees."[12] The water rises above the trees, long and straight *(Sun).* Water has risen above *Sun.* The needle has sunk to the bottom of the sea.

Play Arms Like a Fan

TA CH'U

Play Arms Like a Fan comes from Hexagram 26, *Ta Ch'u,* which means the Taming Power of the Great. The upper trigram is *Ken,* meaning small and hand, and the lower is *Ch'ien,* which means strong, firm, or great. A folding fan, for instance, can be both small and great. The upper nuclear trigram, *Chen,* meaning movement or barnboo, gives more substance to the image of the hands (from *Ken)* moving like a Chinese fan. The lower nuclear trigram, *Tui,* means hurt. One hand is utilized more than the other in the attack against the opponent.

The lower primary trigram, *Ch'ien,* means strong or firm, suggesting the posture of the T'ai Chi Ch'uan practitioner. His two hands rise like the upper nuclear trigram, *Chen. Ken,* the upper trigram, also means mountain. The Image, "Heaven within the mountain," gives the essence of the form: the hands move upward, toward heaven.[13]

Turn Body and Strike Fist to Back

TA KUO

Hexagram 28, *Ta Kuo,* which means Preponderance of the Great, is related to Turn Body and Strike Fist to Back. The upper trigram, *Tui,* denotes lake or to smash. The lower trigram, *Sun,* means either gentle or wind. Both the upper and lower nuclear trigrams are *Ch'ien,* strong or turn. When the nuclear trigrams are changed to three unbroken lines, we have *K'un,* body. Taken together, the trigrams evoke the image of a body turning. The broken line at the top of *Tui* resembles a fist. According to the lines:

> Nine in the third place means:
> The ridgepole sags to the breaking point,

which implies that the fist is thrown back as the body turns.

When he uses this form for self-defense, as the opponent comes from behind, the T'ai Chi player turns around, throws his fist back and delivers a sharp blow to the opponent's head.

> Six at the top means:
> One must go through the water.
> It goes over one's head.

Tui implies water, as well as fist. The fist drops like rain on the opponent's head.

Ta Kuo, the hexagram of this form, is the nuclear hexagram of *Hsiao Kuo,* Hexagram 62, which is related to Needle at Sea Bottom. The lines of *Hsiao Kuo* state:

> Nine in the third place means:
> If one is not extremely careful,
> Somebody may come up from behind and strike him.[14]

Hit Tiger

Hit Tiger originates from Hexagram 42, *I,* which signifies Increase. The upper trigram, *Sun,* denotes gentleness or wind. The lower trigram, *Chen,* for purposes of this analysis signifies movement, foot, and arousing. The upper nuclear trigram is *Ken,* denoting arm, tiger, and temple. The lower nuclear triad is *K'un,* meaning ribs or quietness. Combining the trigrams for arm and movement, the signification is hitting. Adding to this picture the trigram for tiger, we have the T'ai Chi form Hit Tiger.

> Nine at the top means:
> . . . Indeed, someone even strikes him.[15]

The blow is delivered gently, as implied by *Sun* and *K'un.* As the one fist *(Ken)* strikes the temple (again, *Ken*), the other strikes the ribs *(K'un).*

MENG

Kick with Toes

This form and Hexagram 4, *Meng,* share the theme Youthful Folly. The upper trigram, *Ken,* means arm, leg, or mountain. The lower trigram, *K'an,* signifies danger or fetters. The upper nuclear trigram is *K'un,* meaning body or abdomen; the lower nuclear trigram is *Chen,* which means foot and arousing. *Chen* suggests one foot poised to kick. *Ken* suggests that the other foot, like a mountain, is placed solidly on the ground.

The kick is placed below the abdomen, in the genital region (suggested by *K'an,* water). The hands are raised in a block (suggested by the structure of *Ken*) as the kick is delivered. If the opponent catches the foot, the two fists are used to break his hold.

> Nine at the top means:
> In punishing folly
> It does not further one
> To commit transgressions.[16]

These lines, set down to elucidate the hexagram, are appropriate to Kick with Toes, which is used for defensive, not offensive, purposes.

SHIH HO

Hit Opponent's Ears with Fists

Shih Ho, Hexagram 21, is the basis for this form. The meaning of the hexagram is Biting Through. The upper trigram is *Li,* signifying an arrow and suggesting, in its arrangement of lines, two parallel fists: "Strong outside, empty inside." The lower trigram is

Chen, meaning strength or movement. The upper nuclear trigram, *K'an,* signifies ear and danger. The lower nuclear trigram, *Ken,* meaning bow, arm, hand or forehead, combines with *K'an* to intensify the image of striking the ear or forehead.

> Nine at the top means:
> His neck is fastened in the wooden cangue,
> So that his ears disappear.
> Misfortune.[17]

The cangue, an ancient device for punishment, consists of two pieces of wood that grip the neck.

The upper primary trigram, *Li,* and the upper nuclear trigram, *K'an,* together form the image of the bow and arrow. The lower nuclear trigram, *Ken,* can mean legs and in this case indicates a step. The step results in one foot placed forward, bent like a bow, the other behind and straight like an arrow. Thus this form is the bow-and-arrow step of T'ai Chi.

WU WANG

Turn Body and Kick

The form Turn Body and Kick originates from Hexagram 25, *Wu Wang,* Innocence. The upper trigram, *Ch'ien,* means heaven, strength, energy, and to turn. The lower, *Chen,* means movement, foot, and to arouse. The upper nuclear trigram is *Sun,* meaning wind or gentleness. The lower nuclear trigram is *Ken,* which means firmness, leg or mountain.

The hexagram gives a picture of Turn Body and Kick. The player's body (*K'un,* derived by changing the lines of *Ch'ien*) turns (*Ch'ien*) and kicks (*Chen*) gently (*Sun*) like a light wind. *Ken* indicates one leg standing firmly like a mountain. According to the Image given for *Wu Wang,* "Under heaven thunder rolls."[18] When used for self-defense, the natural energy of this movement can be compared to the energy of thunder.

CHUN

Wave Hands Like a Cloud

This form is related to Hexagram 3, *Chun,* Difficulty at the Beginning. The upper trigram, *K'an,* means water, cloud, and wheel. The lower trigram, *Chen,* signifies thunder, wave, or horse. The upper nuclear trigram is *Ken,* meaning hands, arms, or legs. The lower nuclear trigram is *K'un,* indicating the belly or body.

Wave Hands Like a Cloud is built from the composite elements of the hexagram. Cloud comes from *K'an.* The hands *(Ken)* turn *(Chen)* like waves of water *(K'an)* or a wheel *(K'an).* The hands in motion pass across the belly *(K'un),* moving peacefully like clouds floating by in the sky.

> Clouds and thunder:
> The Image of Difficulty at the Beginning.
> Thus the superior man
> Brings order out of confusion.

The posture of the legs in this movement suggests a man mounted on a horse:

> Six in the second place means:
> Difficulties pile up.
> Horse and wagon part.[19]

SHIH

Snake Creeps Down

Hexagram 7, *Shih,* which means the Army, governs Snake Creeps Down. The upper trigram, *K'un,* signifies belly, body, or earth. The lower trigram, *K'an,* means water or snake. The upper nuclear trigram is also *K'un.* The lower nuclear trigram is *Chen,* which means movement and arousing.

The posture of the legs in this movement suggests a snake *(K'an)* creeping on the earth *(K'un).* The player's body is lowered so that the belly *(K'un)* is close to the knees.

The Image of *Shih* says,

> In the middle of the earth is water.

This form involves a kind of retreat from the hand- or foot- blows of the opponent. It is a subtle sinking backward like a strategic retreat by a cautious general.

> Six in the fourth place means:
> The army retreats. No blame.

According to the interpretation of this line: "In face of a superior enemy, with whom it would be hopeless to engage in battle, an orderly retreat is the only correct procedure, because it will save the army from defeat and disintegration. It is by no means a sign of courage or strength to insist upon engaging in a hopeless struggle regardless of circumstances."

The next movement, Golden Cock on One Leg, is more offensive. Thus the purpose of this retreat is to be able to advance later with more success.[20]

Golden Cock on One Leg

CHUNG FU

Golden Cock on One Leg is derived from Hexagram 61, *Chung Fu,* Inner Truth. The upper triad, *Sun,* means chicken or cock (as in the movement Slant Flying) as well as gentleness or wind. *Tui,* the lower trigram, signifies golden. The lower nuclear trigram is *Chen,* foot or arousing, whereas the upper is *Ken,* leg, hand, or mountain. The nuclear trigrams describe this movement: one leg is raised to strike with the knee *(Chen)* and the other is planted firmly on the ground like a mountain *(Ken).* The nuclear triads taken together also suggest that the hands are held above the leg.

LU

High Pat on Horse

This form comes from Hexagram 56, *Lu,* which means the wanderer. *Li,* the upper trigram, signifies "empty inside, strong outside" as well as horse and fire. *Ken,* the lower trigram, means keeping still, mountain, arm, or to pat. The upper nuclear trigram, *Tui,* means oval or to hurt. The lower nuclear trigram, *Sun,* means wind, gentleness, or high. Combining the trigrams we derive High *(Sun)* Pat *(Ken)* on Horse *(Li),* gently *(Sun).* As he works through this movement, the student places one hand slightly above the other so that a space remains between them. Thus the upper hand can suddenly strike the opponent's throat, reaching out in the arc suggested by *Tui,* hurting the opponent as indicated by the same trigram. Meanwhile, the lower hand grabs the combatant's hand *(Ken).*

CHEN

Separate Feet and Kick

The Arousing (Shock, Thunder) is the theme of this form and of Hexagram 51, *Chen.* Both the lower and upper trigrams are *Chen,* meaning to arouse, movement, and foot. The upper nuclear trigram, *K'an,* means water flowing or danger.

The primary trigrams *(Chen)* and the lower nuclear trigram *(Ken)* suggest the hand and leg movements of this form. One foot is poised for kicking *(Chen),* the other is solidly placed *(Ken).* The kick is delivered in a flowing manner, like water *(K'an).*

The Image of this hexagram states:

Thunder repeated: the image of Shock.[21]

Separate Feet and Kick when performed in practice is like flowing water *(K'an).* But in self-defense the movement becomes thunder

(Chen) from the hands and feet. The kick, delivered to the opponent's shin, shocks him like a clap of thunder.

Step Forward and Punch to Opponent's Lower Abdomen

CH'IEN

Step Forward and Punch finds its base in Hexagram 15, *Ch'ien,* which means Modesty. The upper trigram, *K'un,* denotes earth, belly, or abdomen. The lower trigram, *Ken,* means mountain, leg, or arm. The upper nuclear trigram is *Chen* and signifies movement or strength. The lower nuclear trigram is *K'an,* water or danger.

The third line from the bottom of the hexagram, the highest line in *Ken,* signifies a fist. The only strong line in the hexagram, it is placed below the abdomen *(K'un).* The lower nuclear trigram, *K'an,* signifies the genital area, a place of danger if one is attacked.

Taken together the trigrams mean stepping forward to punch below the abdomen.

Modesty is the character of this hexagram. It indicates the gentle, nonaggressive stance of T'ai Chi Ch'uan. This does not mean, of course, that the T'ai Chi practitioner will shy away from force when force is called for.

> Six in the fifth place means:
> . . . It is favorable to attack with force.

Force is used, according to the *I Ching,* "in order to chastise the disobedient."[22]

Fair Lady Works at Shuttles

CHIEH

Hexagram 60, *Chieh,* is related to this form. *Chieh* signifies Limitation. The upper trigram, *K'an,* means water, turn, or wheel. The lower trigram, *Tui,* denotes a fair lady. The upper nuclear trigram is *Ken,* which means mountain, arm, leg, or hand. The lower nuclear trigram is *Chen,* meaning movement, strength, or wood, and suggesting the moving wood of a shuttle. *Chen* also means to cut and left. Combined with *Tui,* which also means right and oval-shaped, these trigrams set the image of a shuttle moving from left to right.

In executing this form, the player's body turns around again and again like a water wheel (suggested by *K'an*). The body turns a total of four times, the number of seasons in the year. The Commentary on *Chieh* includes these appropriate words: "Heaven and earth have their limitations, and the four seasons of the year arise."[23]

The turns in this form must be accomplished smoothly, like flowing water *(K'an).* When used for defense purposes, one hand blocks and the other pushes forward offensively.

FENG

Step Forward, Seven Stars

Step Forward, Seven Stars originates from Hexagram 55, *Feng,* Abundance. The upper trigram, *Chen,* means foot or arousing. The lower trigram, *Li,* signifies fire, sun, or eye. The upper nuclear trigram is *Tui,* which means to hurt. The lower nuclear trigram is *Sun,* gentleness or strength.

One foot, in accordance with *Chen,* is aroused and ready to kick. The one broken line of *Tui* symbolizes the two fists before the chest. *Sun* means that the motions in this movement are executed gently. *Li* signifies the sun, the star of our solar system. When the Judgment reads, "Be like the sun at midday," it refers to the two fists in the middle of the chest.

> Six in the second place means:
> . . . That the polestars can be seen at noon.

The polestars are a cluster of seven stars, and their mention in this statement relates the hexagram to the movement, Step Forward, Seven Stars.

The lower nuclear trigram, *Sun,* can also mean forward and backward. "It is advance and retreat." The Commentary on the hexagram points out the waxing and waning flow of events in nature: "When the sun stands at midday, it begins to set." This leads to Ride Tiger to the Mountain, a form of retreat.[24]

CHIEN

Ride Tiger to the Mountain

Chien, Hexagram 53, is the basis in the *I Ching* for Ride Tiger to the Mountain. The hexagram means Development. The upper trigram, *Sun,* signifies gentleness and wind. The lower trigram, *Ken,* means mountain, arm, leg, and tiger. The upper nuclear trigram is *Li,* meaning arrow, and the lower nuclear trigram is *K'an,* meaning bow. The broken line of *Sun* symbolizes the student's two legs. With the meanings mountain and tiger from *Ken,* the two trigrams together yield this T'ai Chi form.

WEI CHI

Turn Body and Do Lotus Kick

This movement is taken from Hexagram 64, *Wei Chi,* Before Completion. The upper trigram, *Li,* means sun, fire, and eyes. The lower trigram, *K'an,* signifies water, wheel, turn, and devil. The upper nuclear trigram is also *K'an* and the lower is, again, *Li.* Turn *(K'an)* the whole body like a wheel *(K'an).*

> Nine in the fourth place means:
> Perseverance brings good fortune.
> Remorse disappears.
> Shock, thus to discipline the Devil's Country.[25]

The shock refers to the kick, delivered to the middle section of the opponent's body. *K'an* also means kidney, which is known in this Taoist system as "the Devil's Country."

Shoot Tiger

HSIEH

Deliverance, the meaning of Hexagram 40, *Hsieh,* is the rationale for Shoot Tiger. The upper trigram, *Chen,* signifies movement, strength, thunder, and foot. The lower trigram, *K'an,* means water, wheel, bow, rain, and danger. The lower nuclear trigram is *Li,* meaning arrow.

We have, by combining *Li* and *K'an,* the image of the bow and arrow. *Chen,* when inverted, becomes *Ken,* which has the meanings of tiger and arm. And these trigrams give the image of shooting the tiger. Two fists are pressed forward (from *Chen,* movement). *Li* signifies that the arrows are aimed at the opponent's temple and ribs. According to the Commentary on the Decision of *Hsieh:* "Danger (from *K'an*) produces movement *(Chen).* Through movement one escapes danger: this is deliverence."[26]

Circle Fist

TING

Circle Fist is taken from Hexagram 50, Ting, the Caldron. The upper trigram, *Li,* means weapon, eyes, and suggests the aphorism, "Strong outside, empty inside." The lower trigram, *Sun,* signifies wood, gentleness, and strength. The upper nuclear trigram is *Tui,* which means smash, hurt, or right. The lower nuclear trigram is *Ch'ien.*

The fists of this form are suggested by the top line of *Tui.* The lower trigram, *Sun,* denotes the two feet standing firmly. The player circles his fist to smash *(Tui)* the opponent's head *(Ch'ien).*

At the end of the second section, the form Cross Hands, based on Hexagram 36, *Ming I,* is repeated. The return to *Ming I,* Darkening of the Light, means that this section of movements can be compared to the cycle of the sun as it moves from one horizon to the next. To conclude the section Form 1, the Beginning of the T'ai Chi Ch'uan, derived from *Chin* (the sun rising), is repeated. The whole cycle of movements can then be repeated from the beginning, as the sun rising and setting once more.

CHIN

MING I

V. T'AI CHI CH'UAN USED FOR
SELF-DEFENSE

I have discovered that there are many misconceptions about the use of T'ai Chi Ch'uan for self-defense. Westerners usually regard T'ai Chi as only a health exercise, or else they assume that it is simply a variation of Karate or Judo. The T'ai Chi Ch'uan system does contain self-defense forms which originated in the Taoist competition with the Buddhist form of Shiao-lin boxing. This competition is spoken of in many of the older legends and stories from Chinese history.

Self-defense naturally involves rapid hand and leg movements that are quite a bit faster than the movements used when T'ai Chi is practiced alone. Although this is true, the spirit of self-defense in T'ai Chi is identical to the spirit used in executing the forms. It is relaxed and smooth, without anxiety or pride. Its particular flavor is best exemplified by the *I Ching* aphorism, "Only through the divine can one hurry without haste and reach the goal without walking."[1] Even in self-defense one must learn to abide in the Tao.

After becoming skilled in the practice of the forms, the next step is to learn to push hands. This involves the four fundamental forms: Push Up, Pull Back, Press Forward, and Push Forward. Pushing hands reinforces or corrects the student's execution of the forms, at the same time that it is the first step in the practice of self-defense. It makes the player more balanced and pliable. One learns the opponent's intentions from actual contact with him.

SINGLE PUSH HAND

Two opponents stand face to face, two steps apart. Each steps forward on his right foot and raises his right arm so that the opponents' wrists touch with palms turned inward to the chest. Then a circular movement is transacted by the arms as they move forward and backward with the wrists still touching. The left feet are then brought forward and the left hands perform a similar movement.

DOUBLE PUSH HANDS

When the second opponent *(B)* raises his right arm to resist the first opponent *(A)*, *A* places his palms on *B*'s right arm and pushes forward against *B*'s chest (Fig. 65). *B* raises his arms with *A*'s palms still adhering to his right arm. *B* is now ready to counterattack.

A pushes forward and shifts his weight to the right foot and puts his left hand on his own right wrist, pressing forward against *B* (Fig. 66). *B* turns his body, shifts to left foot, raises his right arm, elbow touching *A*'s arm and then pulls to the left side. The left hand pushes *A*'s elbow and the right hand pushes his wrist, continuing to push up and press forward.

When *A* is pressed by *B*'s movements forward, he shifts his weight to the left leg, raising his right arm, with his elbow touching *B*'s arm

Fig. 65   Fig. 66

(Fig. 67). At the same time he sinks back slightly with his elbow turned to the left rear to neutralize *B*'s force. Then *A*'s right hand moves down and around *B*'s right hand and leads it to the side. *A*'s right hand crosses and pushes against the wrist while the left hand pushes the elbow or forearm (Fig. 68).

Then push forward as in Fig. 65 and press forward as in Fig. 66.

MOVING DOUBLE PUSH HANDS

In the previous Push Hand forms, the lower body remains fixed, while the upper body moves back and forth. In Moving Push Hands, the hand movements continue while the legs move backward and forward in coordination with the hand movements.

A and *B* push hands as described in Double Push Hands. Continuing these movements, *A* takes one step forward, and at the same time *B* takes one step backward (*A* advances toward *B* while *B* retreats). This is repeated, each time adding an additional step. Three steps are sufficient.

Fig. 67   Fig. 68

Ta Lu

The next practice step is called *Ta Lu*. At the same time that *A* makes one step forward and another sideward, *B* steps backward and retreats one step to the side. Thus, all four corners of an imaginary square in which the opponents practice are covered by their steps. Besides the hand movements Push Up, Pull Back, and Press Forward, *Ta Lu* also includes other movements. All together *Ta Lu* consists of eight moves which correspond to the eight trigrams of the *I Ching*.

When these self-defense forms have been mastered, the student can begin to learn Hand-to-Hand Combat, also known as Separate Hand. This is a complete system of hand combat which consists of eighty-eight distinct movements with variations, utilizing each form of the T'ai Chi Ch'uan. Several of these movements are demonstrated in Figs. 69–74. The step-by-step mastery of T'ai Chi for self-defense is comparable to learning the *I Ching*, which precedes from understanding the eight trigrams to mastery of the sixty-four hexagrams with their 384 lines.

Needle at Sea Bottom (Fig. 69)

If the opponent strikes with his fist or holds your wrist, grasp his wrist and pull it down, using the intrinsic force and weight of your trunk and legs. He will lose his balance and fall forward. If he resists or lifts his arms upward, use Play Arms Like a Fan to lift his arms and strike his waist with your left palm.

Snake Creeps Down (Fig. 70)

If the opponent strikes with his fist high, Snake Creeps Down can be used to escape the blow.

GOLDEN COCK ON ONE LEG (FIGS. 71, 72, 73)

After retreating from the opponent with the form Snake Creeps Down, one of these variations of Golden Cock on One Leg can be used to counterattack. In Fig. 71 the left arm lifts the opponent's elbow while the right knee strikes his lower abdomen. In Figs. 72 and 73 the right arm grasps the opponent's arm to hold him in range while the left hand thrusts at his throat. Simultaneously, in Fig. 72 the right foot kicks the opponent's leg, while in Fig. 73 the right knee is used against his lower abdomen.

STEP FORWARD AND PUNCH (FIG. 74)

This form can also be adapted to avoid the opponent's high punch. The left arm raises the opponent's arm at the elbow while the right fist punches his abdomen. At the same time as the punch is executed, the step is taken to increase the punching arm's forward thrust.

Fig. 69   Fig. 70

Fig. 71

Fig. 72

Fig. 73

Fig. 74

VI. TAOIST MEDITATION AND
T'AI CHI CH'UAN

The highest goal in Taoism is to reach a state of consciousness which transcends the bonds of mortality that cramp ordinary existence. This state is the Tao. The achievement of the Tao can be realized only after a long process of insight and concentration. The subtle process of Taoist meditation is exceedingly complex and varies from one master to another. Accuracy and resultant progress depend on the degree of enlightenment of the master who supervises the process.

Taoist meditation can be thought of as an alchemical procedure. It involves the refinement of one psychic substance into another. The process begins with *ching,* or sexual energy. *Ching* is converted into another substance, *chi,* when it is combined with the breath in a certain way. The purification of *chi* results in its transformation to *shen,* or spirit. In the last stage *shen* is converted to *shu,* or emptiness. T'ai Chi Ch'uan gives an outer image of the inner transformations of Taoist meditation. The T'ai Chi movements are paradigms of the inner processes that take place in Taoist alchemy.

When a metal is to be transformed by alchemy, it is usually heated for a period of time in a special flask. The heating process is repeated several times. Then the purified substance is passed to another flask where it is transformed in a new way. A bellows is used frequently by the alchemist to regulate the temperature and intensity of the fire.

The body of the student of Taoist meditation can be compared to the alchemist's laboratory. The psychic centers, or spiritual organs, of the body have the function of the flasks in alchemical distillation. The breath of the meditator can be compared to the bellows and the psychic fluid to the elixir which is passed from one flask to another in the laboratory.

In our bodily laboratory, then, we have twelve flasks, or psychic centers. In Taoist symbolism these centers are referred to as months of the year or constellations of the zodiac. Each one of these points can be represented by a hexagram of the *I Ching*. For instance, the point at the base of the spine, known as *wei lu* or the Gate of the Tail, corresponds to the hexagram *Fu;* the psychic center located in the brain and known as *ni wan* corresponds to the hexagram *Ko*.

As meditation begins the *ching,* or sexual energy, is moved upward to a point about an inch and a half below the navel. This may be compared to the process of heating a caldron on a stove. The point is known as the *tan tien*. At the *tan tien* the first purification cycle begins. This cycle is known as the Lesser Heavenly Circulation and is elegantly described by the first T'ai Chi Ch'uan movement.

From an erect position, with knees slightly bent, arms at sides with palms facing backward, both hands are slowly raised to the level of the shoulders and then slowly pressed down to the original position, as though an invisible force were pulling them up and down. As the hands are raised, the breath is drawn in and as they are lowered, it is exhaled. In this movement the *chi* is experienced as rising from the *tan tien* and then descending back to it as the arms are raised and lowered. When breathing in, the *chi* moves up in the front of the body; when breathing out, it moves down. This up-and-down movement is sometimes poetically referred to as the union of *Li* and *K'an,* fire and water. *K'an,* which means water, refers to the region of the lower abdomen, which is known as the Seat of Water. It also refers to the psychic center of this region. *Li,* on the other hand, which means fire, refers to the region of the heart and its corresponding spiritual center. Passion, which springs from the heart region, can appropriately be compared to fire and this region is often known as the Seat of Fire. Thus, the first T'ai Chi movement describes a process of ascent and descent between these two regions until the elixir slips back into the *tan tien*. The subtle substance is now ready for its next step of purification, known as the Greater Heavenly Circulation.

The Greater Heavenly Circulation is a purification cycle that passes the *chi* through all the psychic centers. *Ching* has already been transformed to *chi* by its admixture with breath during the Lesser Heavenly Current. The *chi* must now pass through the two main channels: one in front of the body, known as *Jen Mu* or the "involuntary course," and one in the back called *Tu Mu* or the "controlled course." *Tu Mu* is comprised of the psychic centers known respectively as *wei lu* (at the tip of the spine), *shun fu* (slightly below the middle of the spine), *hsuan shu* (in the middle of the spine), *chai chi* (slightly above the middle of the spine), *t'ao tao* (below the neck), *yu chen* (in the back of the head), *ni wan* (crown of the head), and *ming t'ung* (between the eyebrows). *Tu Mu* ends at the upper lip. *Jen Mu* begins in the lower lip and passes through *t'an chung* (in the chest), *chung huan* (above the navel), *shen chueh* (in the navel), and *ch'i hai* (about three inches below the navel).

The Greater Heavenly Circulation is captured in the Tai Chi Ch'uan form Step Back and Repulse Monkey. In this form the movement of the *chi* is described by the movement of the player's hands. The right hand drops to the region of the thigh, moves back and rises to the top of the head, and then is pushed forward and down, returning to the starting point. The left hand describes the same movements. However, when the right hand is at the top of the head, the left hand is in the thigh region. The relation of the two hands can be thought of as two diametrically opposed spokes of a wheel, while the movement of the wheel itself signifies the orbiting of the *chi* through the Greater Heavenly Circulation.

These are not the only orbits used in meditation for purposes of purification of the elixir. T'ai Chi Ch'uan describes several other orbits. For instance, a series of forms beginning with White Crane Spreads Wings illustrates a related but more extensive movement than the Lesser Heavenly Current. As the student executes the White Crane movement, the right hand guides the *chi* from the *tan tien* in the abdomen to the *ming t'ung*, the center between the eyes. Then the right hand brings the *chi* down again to the abdomen. The circulation of *chi* is continued in the next form, Brush Knee and Push, where the *chi* is brought down below the abdomen to the genital region and then up again until it reaches the throat center. The *chi* is brought down again, in the form Needle at Sea Bottom, to the genital region. The *chi* is then raised as the hands move apart in Play Arms Like a Fan. In this form *chi* is brought back through the *ming t'ung*, through the *ni wan* to the top of the head and then down again.

Another orbit of the *chi* is demonstrated by the movement Wave

Hands Like a Cloud. In meditation this orbit is conceived within a plane inside the belly. In the T'ai Chi form the left hand guides the *chi* from the upper left down to the right side of the body. Then the right hand starts from the lower left and moves in a graceful circle to the upper right, then down again to the right.

Whereas Wave Hands Like a Cloud describes an unusual orbit of the *chi* in the front of the belly, the form Fair Lady Works at Shuttles describes a similarly unusual orbit which circulates from the front of the belly to the back. Then the orbit itself pivots on its axis and the *chi* takes a similar but opposite course throughout the body. In the form itself there are two pivots to the right and two to the left. The orbit of the *chi* is elliptical and turns on an axis which is tilted in a northeasterly angle to the vertical.

From the upper left, the left hand sweeps downward to the right, describing the *chi* moving downward in the arc in the front of the belly. The body then pivots to the left, indicating an epicycle formed after the *chi* passes into the base of the dorsal region. The left hand, now at the right bottom, then sweeps upward and to the left, retracing the original arc of the *chi* back through the familiar orbit. The right hand is then pushed forward, bringing the *chi* down to the right as the body then pivots to the left and the right hand then channels the *chi* upward to the left. In the next two parts of the form, the body pivots to the right and the *chi,* in general, passes up through the top of the head, makes its little epicycle and passes down again. This passage is signified by the hands moving up, the body pivoting, and the hands moving down again.

Besides demonstrating the circulation of *chi,* T'ai Chi Ch'uan is related to classic Chinese sitting meditation in a number of ways. Both require keeping the torso erect but relaxed, the head erect, the neck straight, the arms and legs curved, and the shoulders down with the arms relaxed. The mind, in both cases, must be clear and still. Both require "right effort," a kind of effortless concentration free of goals or pride. In T'ai Chi the body moves outside and is still inside; in sitting meditation there must be stillness within and without. Breathing is an essential part of T'ai Chi and meditation; but in T'ai Chi breathing is assisted by the body's movement, whereas in meditation the breath is controlled solely by the mind.

T'ai Chi Ch'uan can be considered a kind of preparatory exercise for meditation, although, of course, it can be studied for a variety of other reasons. It disciplines the body, teaches relaxation and clearheadedness, accustoms the student to regulated breathing, and demonstrates the circulation of *chi* by a method far more close to the real event of meditation than looking at diagrams or hearing oral descriptions. More than that, T'ai Chi Ch'uan gives something of the spirit of meditation, a spirit which, in our overactive, anxiety-ridden lives, we seldom taste in day-to-day living—a spirit which promises a glimpse of peace beyond the scope of our present imagination or our ordinary understanding of the world.

VII. THE WAXING AND WANING OF CH'IEN AND K'UN AS APPLIED TO THE PRACTICE OF T'AI CHI CH'UAN

The flow and accumulation of energy in the body during the practice of T'ai Chi Ch'uan can be represented in an accurate and enlightening way by means of the cycle of twelve hexagrams known as the "Waxing and Waning of Ch'ien and K'un." First discovered by the philosopher Meng Hsi during the early Han period, this cycle has been widely used for theoretical purposes in several different fields of Chinese traditional knowledge, including acupuncture, meditation, and the calendar.

The cycle itself is fairly simple to describe, the ideas of "waxing" and "waning" having to do with the orderly increase and decrease of the number of unbroken (*yang*) lines in the hexagrams involved. The cycle may be thought of as starting from the Hexagram 24, *Fu* ䷗ , which has a *yang* line in the lowest place, and all of its remaining lines are *yin*. At later stages in the cycle, the *yang* lines move successively higher into the hexagrams, and the lines below them remain *yang*. Thus after *Fu*, the next hexagram is Hexagram 19, *Lin* ䷒ , in which the bottom two lines are *yang*. The next is Hexagram 11, *T'ai* ䷊ , with *yang* lines in its first three places, and so on. By continuing this increase in the number of *yang* lines, one soon comes to Hexagram 1, Ch'ien ䷀ , all of whose lines are *yang*. This completes the "waxing" part of the cycle, after which the "waning" begins.

The first hexagram in the "waning" part of the cycle is Hexagram 44, *Kou* ䷫ in which one *yin* line appears on the

bottom. Next is Hexagram 33, *Tun* ☴ , which has two *yin*
lines. This phase of the cycle continues until Hexagram 2, *K'un*
☷ , is obtained, in which all the lines are *yin*, completing
the waning.

With a bit of imagination, it is not difficult to see how this
pattern of hexagrams can be used to give an accurate account
of the regular cyclic processes of nature, such as the phases of
the moon and seasons of the year. What is perhaps less ob-
vious, but no less useful once the idea is understood, is to
apply the same principles to the description of cyclic processes
within the body. In fact, the flow of energy during the practice
of the T'ai Chi Ch'uan form is a particularly good example of
such an application.

To begin with, it is sufficient to consider the very first movement of the form, in which the arms are raised while the knees
are slightly straightened, and then lowered to the sides as the
knees are bent once again. The movements of the limbs in this
form are designed to guide the flow of the *ch'i* (vital energy)
from the feet up the spine to the top of the head and then
down the front of the body to the abdomen. To describe this
flow of vital energy, the waxing and waning of Ch'ien and K'un
is quite appropriate, for each hexagram in the cycle indicates
the progression of the energy to a certain part of the body. *Fu*
represents the very beginning, in which the energy rises from
the soles of the feet. *Ch'ien* represents the point at which the
knees are straight and the energy has risen up through the
spinal column all the way to the head. *K'un* represents the
outcome of the lowering, in which the energy has moved
down to the abdomen.

The following descriptions indicate the significance of each
of the hexagrams in the cycle for the energy flow.

24   Fu

Fu/Return

The upper trigram is *K'un*, The Receptive, earth, a pliable body.
The lower trigram is *Chen*, The Arousing, thunder, wood, foot.
The nuclear trigrams are both *K'un*.

With three *K'un* and one *Chen*, earth and wood, we may think of a tree deeply rooted in the earth.

The T'ai Chi Ch'uan student stands firmly like a tree well-rooted in the ground. His torso is pliant and resilient. He stands like a bottom-weighted doll and cannot be overturned. The energy is in his feet and will begin to rise up to the spinal cord.*

The Sequence says: "Things cannot be destroyed once and for all. When what is above is completely split apart, it returns below. Hence there follows the hexagram of Return."* While *Fu* is here presented as the first hexagram in this cycle, it must be remembered that it follows the last hexagram in the previous cycle, *K'un*. Mention is also made here of *Po*/Splitting Apart, which precedes *K'un*, and is the opposite of *Fu*.

The hexagram designates December and January, the winter solstice. Trees and grass are bare of leaves although their roots are beginning to stir. It is the midnight of quietness and recovery of life. The *yin*, negative, is waning and will soon be gone. The *yang*, positive, is reappearing. The Inner Elixir is beginning to sprout.

The Commentary on the Decision says: "'Return has success.' The firm returns. Movement and action through devotion. Therefore, 'Going out and coming in without error.' . . . This is the course of heaven."[1] By devotion (from the trigram *K'un*) to the practice of T'ai Chi Ch'uan the student achieves success. Going out and coming in refer to the opposite nature of the T'ai Chi movements: up and down, back and forth, left and right and breathing in and out. The course of heaven represents the circulation of the *ch'i.*

It is said in Chapter 40 of the *Tao Te Ching*:

> Return is the movement of the Tao.
> Pliant is the application of the Tao.[2]

Thus T'ai Chi Ch'uan is the Taoist exercise which is performed in a cycle which completes itself and then continues (returns).

When the first *yang* line increases to the second, the hexagram becomes Hexagram 19, *Lin*/Approach.

19   Lin

Lin/Approach

> The upper trigram is *k'un*, The Receptive, earth.
> The lower trigram is *Tui*, The Joyous, Lake.
> The nuclear trigrams are *K'un* and *Chên*, The Arousing, Thunder.

The hexagram *Lin* means approach. In the previous hexagram, *Fu*, the *yang* line energy in the first line is far below the ground like a root. In the hexagram *Lin* the *yang* lines increase to two. In the Commentary on the Decision it says, "The firm penetrates and grows."[3] The "firm" refers to the *yang* power or energy represented by the first two lines of the hexagram. This energy, below the surface in *Fu*, has begun to grow by virtue of the penetration of the water, represented by the trigram *Tui*, into the earth, represented by the trigram *K'un*. This moisture provides nourishment to the roots and ultimately to the wood, both indicated by the lower nuclear trigram *Chen*, which can then grow more quickly.

The Commentary on the Decision continues:

> Joyous and devoted . . .
> "Great success through correctness:" this is
> the course of heaven.[4]

By devotion to the careful and correct practice of the forms, the T'ai Chi student can achieve a healthy body, through which he can experience greater enjoyment of his life. However, *Tui*, which means enjoyment, can also mean hurt or injury, and so the student is warned against careless practice of the exercise which could lead to injury.

"This is the course of heaven" means that this energy, which has begun to grow, will penetrate into the spinal cord and enter the "Greater Heavenly Circulation."

The time represented is January–February, the twelfth month.

When the two *yang* lines increase to three, the hexagram becomes Hexagram 11, *T'ai*/Peace.

T'ai/Peace

The upper trigram is *K'un*, The Receptive, earth.
The lower trigram is *Ch'ien*, The Creative, heaven.
The nuclear trigrams are *Chên*, The Arousing, Thunder and *Tui*, The Joyous, Lake.

T'ai means peaceful, penetration or harmony and is a time of flowering. This is the idea of the T'ai Chi Ch'uan. One practices without strain or intensity and feels peaceful and relaxed.

The second meaning of the hexagram *T'ai* is penetration. After practicing, one feels the blood circulating and the breathing penetrates the whole body, even to the fingertips and toes.

According to the character of the upper trigram, *K'un* means pliable and devoted. The lower trigram, *Ch'ien*, is strong and firm, which indicates that one should practice T'ai Chi Ch'uan with the weight in the lower part of the body. The lower body is strong and firm. The upper body is pliable and devoted. The Commentary on the Decision states: "Strength is within and devotion without."[5] This indicates that the T'ai Chi Ch'uan practitioner is gaining mastery. He is firm inside and soft outside, like cotton wrapped around steel.

"In the way heaven and earth unite, and all beings come into union. Upper and lower unite and they are of one will."[6] Through circulation of the *ch'i* the head and the lower body are united. In the T'ai Chi Classics it says that each movement should be light and nimble, but most importantly it must be unified.

If we study the upper trigram *k'un*, the three lines broken in the middle indicate that the breathing can reach down to the abdomen without any hindrance. In the lower trigram, *Ch'ien*, the three unbroken lines indicate the solidity of the lower part of the body, and also the spinal cord. Thus the *yang* force has now risen half way up the spinal cord.

When the bottom three *yang* lines increase to four, the next hexagram is Hexagram 34, *Ta Chuang*/The Power of the Great.

34   Ta Chuang

Ta Chuang/The Power of the Great

The upper trigram is *Chen*, The Arousing, Thunder.
The lower trigram is *Ch'ien*, The Creative, Heaven, strong.
The nuclear trigrams are *Tui*, the Joyous, Lake, and *Ch'ien*.

The structure of this hexagram is very strong. It is analagous to the spinal cord of the T'ai Chi student.

According to the T'ai Chi Ch'uan Classics, when you stand still every part of your body is tranquil; when you move, the Intrinsic Energy moves to the back of the body and centers in the spinal cord.

The individual lines of the hexagram refer to the way in which the T'ai Chi Ch'uan practitioner masters his art.

The first line says, "Power in the toes. Continuing brings misfortune."[7] This refers to the continuing movement of the T'ai Chi Ch'uan which does not remain in one position for long, but shifts to a new position in order to maintain perfect balance. The power cannot be only in the toes, but must go to the whole foot to assure stability.

The third line says, "The inferior man works through power. The superior man does not act thus . . . A goat butts against a hedge and gets its horn entangled."[8] The T'ai Chi Ch'uan practitioner does not use strength in his movements for health or self defense. He is pliable and yielding, but strong within.

The fourth line says, "The hedge opens, there is no entanglement."[9] If the T'ai Chi practitioner is yielding, he gives way under attack and thus saves himself from entanglement.

The sixth line warns the T'ai Chi practitioner against the use of strength. The text says, "A goat butts against a hedge. It cannot go backward, it cannot go forward."[10]

Thus the message of this hexagram is that even if the T'ai Chi player possesses great strength he should not use it, for it tempts disaster. The T'ai Chi master maintains a soft and humble exterior even though he has great strength hidden within.

Lao Tzu advises this principle of action in the *Tao Te Ching*:

> The weakest things in the world can overmatch the strongest things in the world.
> Nothing in the world can be compared to water for its weak and yielding nature; yet in attacking the hard and strong nothing proves better than it.[11]

Lao Tzu also applies this idea to the health aspects of T'ai Chi Ch'uan, as he says:

> Man when living is soft and tender;
> When dead he is hard and tough.[12]

This hexagram represents the second month (March–April). When the four *yang* lines increase to five the new hexagram is Hexagram 43, *Kuai*/Resoluteness.

43   Kuai

Kuai/Resoluteness

The upper trigram is *Tui*, The Joyous, Lake, Injury.
The lower trigram is *Ch'ien*, The Creative, Heaven, Strength.
The nuclear trigrams are both *Ch'ien*.

The Hexagram *Kuai* means resoluteness. The structure of this hexagram represents a joyous and peaceful mind and an energetic body.

It is said in the T'ai Chi Ch'uan classic that through long practice, energy can be accumulated. The body becomes strong physically and the mind becomes resolute and thus acts with joy.

The Commentary on the Decision says, "Strong and joyous—this means resolute and harmonious."[13]

When T'ai Chi Ch'uan is performed consistently over a long period of time, or resolutely and with *joy*, one's mind and body become harmonious. Thus resolution is characterized by patience, perseverance and determination but is not anxious.

The third line of the hexagram says:

> To be powerful in the cheekbones
> Brings misfortune.[14]

This means that strength should be on the inside and not exhibited on the outside.

The same idea is found in Chapter 68 of Lao Tzu's *Tao Te Ching*:

> The best soldier is not warlike.
> A skillful fighter is not angry.[15]

In this hexagram the *yang* lines have continued to increase. The energy continues to rise along the spinal cord up to the head (heaven) like the evaporation of the waters of the lake (*Tui*). This phenomenon is described in the Image:

> The lake has risen up to heaven,
> The image of Break-through.[16]

When the remaining *yin* line is pushed out, there will be six *yang* lines, forming the Hexagram *Ch'ien*.

1   Ch'ien

Ch'ien/The Creative

The upper trigram is *Ch'ien*, The Creative, Heaven, head.
The lower trigram is *Ch'ien*.
The nuclear trigrams are both *Ch'ien*.

This hexagram is composed of six *yang* lines. In Wilhelm's translation of the *I Ching*, it says, "These unbroken lines stand for primal power, which is light-giving, active and strong of the spirit."[17]

When the T'ai Chi Ch'uan master reaches this level, his mind is filled with spirit, his body is filled with energy, his bones are filled with marrow and he is pliable and resilient like steel.

The Image of the hexagram says:

> The movement of heaven is strong and regular.
> The superior man fortifies himself unceasingly.[18]

In many activities growth and progress depend on continued practice. This is especially true of T'ai Chi Ch'uan. The third line of the hexagram says:

> All day long the superior man is creatively active.
> At nightfall his mind is still beset with cares.[19]

This means that the T'ai Chi student should practice both in the day and at night. According to the T'ai Chi Classics, after many years of such practice, the body and mind are ultimately guided by the spirit. If one overemphasizes the use of energy, he will stagnate. If one does not use up the energy, it becomes pure vitality. In its highest degree T'ai Chi Ch'uan becomes pure and resilient, and uses the spirit. There are several names for this level. The Taoists call it "Chen Jen,"[20] the true man. The Confucians call it "Ta Jen,"[21] the great man, and the Buddhists call it "Chin Kang,"† literally meaning strong like gold or diamond, that is, indestructible. A man like this is unconquerable. Lao Tzu describes this man in Chapter 50 of the *Tao Te Ching*:

> He who knows how to live can travel in the
>   wilderness
> Without fearing rhinoceros or tiger.
> He will not be wounded by weapons,
> In him rhinoceroses can find no opportunity
>   to thrust their horns,
> And tigers no chance to use their claws.
> Why is this so?
> Because he is not vulnerable.[22]

This same idea is also found in the T'ai Chi Classics where it says:

> One can feel even a feather on his body,
> Or the landing of a fly.[23]

With the Hexagram *Ch'ien* the energy has reached the head or the 'Yu Chen.' All the lines are *yang*. But this condition will not last. When a *yin* line enters in the first place, the hexagram is Hexagram 44, *Kou*/Coming to Meet, and the waning part of the cycle begins.

44   Kou

Kou/Coming to Meet

The upper trigram is *Ch'ien*, The Creative, Heaven.
The lower trigram is *Sun*, The Gentle, The Penetrating,
    Wind.
The nuclear trigrams are both *Ch'ien*.

The hexagram *Kou* means Coming to Meet. The last hexagram, *Ch'ien*, with six *yang* lines, is full of the light power.

However, like the moon, once it has become full, it will begin to wane. *Kou* indicates the beginning of the waning part of the cycle.

The hexagram *Kou* represents the fifth month, June–July, and the time of the Summer Solstice. From this point on the days become shorter and the nights become longer.

The Commentary on the Decision says, "The Weak advances to meet the Firm."[24] "Weak" refers to the one *yin* line entering at the bottom of the hexagram, which is encountering the "Firm" or *yang* lines which compose the remainder of the hexagram. This *yin* force will continue to grow in the succeeding hexagrams in the cycle.

"He comes to meet with his horns,"[25] is the sixth line of the hexagram. Horns refer to the head or crown, which is the point to which the *ch'i* has risen in the waxing portion of the cycle. It is the point, described in works on acupuncture and meditation, where the *Tu Mo*, or channel of control (*yang*), meets with the *Jen Mo*, the channel of function (*yin*). In the T'ai Chi Ch'uan Classics this is described as the point at which the energy begins to descend. If the spinal cord is held correctly, erect and in the middle, then the *ch'i*, having reached the head, will become saliva and go down to the *tan t'ien*.

When the *yin* force advances to the second line, the hexagram becomes Hexagram 33, *Tun*/Retreat.

33   Tun

Tun/Retreat

The upper trigram is *Ch'ien*, The Creative, Heaven.
The lower trigram is *Ken*, Keeping Still, Mountain.
The nuclear trigrams are *Ch'ien* and *Sun*, The Gentle, Wind.

This hexagram means retreat or withdraw. The forces of light (*yang*) are retreating before the steady advance of the forces of darkness (*yin*). It is the opposite of the hexagram 34, *Ta Chuang*, which means advance and was seen earlier in the cycle. In the calendar it represents the sixth month, July–August, when summer has already begun to fade.

In the Commentary on the Decision it says, "Retreat. Success: this means that success lies in retreating."[26] In some situations retreat is the appropriate course of action; recognizing the time for retreat will bring success. In performing the T'ai Chi Ch'uan form it is proper to retreat when the *ch'i* has begun its descent into the *tan t'ien*, for then, the growth of the vitality will take place.

In this book, in Chapter IV, p. 60, *Tun* is associated with the form "Step Back and Repulse Monkey." This move represents the physical retreat of the body. In the "Waxing and Waning of Ch'ien and K'un" retreat refers to the movement of the mind and *ch'i*.

When the *yin* has advanced to the third line the hexagram becomes Hexagram 12, *P'i*/Standstill.

P'i/Standstill

The upper trigram is *Ch'ien*, The Creative, Heaven.
The lower trigram is *K'un*, The Receptive, Earth.
The nuclear trigrams are *Sun*, The Gentle, Penetrating, Wind, and *Ken*, Keeping Still, Mountain.

This hexagram means Standstill. The trigrams *Ch'ien* and *K'un* move in opposite directions in contrast to Hexagram II, *T'ai*/Peace, where the trigrams move towards each other. This movement results in standstill, and is reinforced by the meaning of the lower nuclear trigram, *Ken*, which means Keeping Still.

"The great departs; the small approaches."[27] This line from the Judgment describes the departure of *yang* ("the great") and the approach of *yin* ("the small"). In the calendar it refers to the seventh month, August–September, the beginning of autumn.

The second line of the hexagram says, "The Standstill serves to help the great man to attain success."[28] In spite of the continuing advance of the *yin* power the situation is still favorable. It is like autumn when many leaves have fallen from the trees. As long as their roots remain alive, they will be able to grow again in the spring. In the performance of T'ai Chi Ch'uan, the *ch'i* must continue to descend and reach the *tan t'ien* before it will be ready to ascend again.

When the *yin* power reaches the fourth line, the hexagram becomes Hexagram 20, *Kuan*/Contemplation.

Kuan/Contemplation

20   Kuan

The upper trigram is *Sun*, The Gentle, Penetrating, Wind.
The lower trigram is *K'un*, The Receptive, Earth.
The nuclear trigrams are *Ken*, Keeping Still, Mountain, and *K'un*.

This hexagram means contemplation and observation. The *yin* power has continued to increase until only the top two lines remain *yang*. It is the time of the eighth month, September–October.

The dual meaning of the hexagram *Kuan*, observation and contemplation, can be directly related to the practice of T'ai Chi Ch'uan. Contemplation refers to the inner process in which the *ch'i* sinks further down on its way to the *tan t'ien*. The lower trigram *K'un*, also the lower nuclear trigram, represents this place. Observation, on the other hand, directs the student to the outer aspects of the exercise. He observes the correctness of his form and notices if the approach of any opponents threaten his position.

The following lines from the Ta Chuan, describing Hexagram 16, *Yü*/Enthusiasm, give an example of the importance of observation in the practice of T'ai Chi Ch'uan.

> The superior man knows what is hidden and what
>   is evident.
> He knows weakness, he knows strength as well.
> Hence the myriads look up to him.[29]

Thus the T'ai Chi master knows if the enemy is weak or strong, and can achieve success by defeating him. This will cause many people, especially his students, to look up to him.

When only one *yang* line remains, the hexagram becomes Hexagram 23, *Po*/Splitting Apart.

Po/Splitting Apart

The upper trigram is *Ken*, Keeping Still, Mountain.
The lower trigram is *K'un*, The Receptive, Earth.
The nuclear trigrams are both *K'un*.

The hexagram *Po* means decline, decay and ruin. In the calendar it represents the ninth month, October–November. All the lines have become *yin*, except for the top line. The text for this line reads: "There is still a large fruit uneaten."

The "large fruit" refers to the one *yang* line remaining at the top of the hexagram. Farmers often save the best fruits to provide seed for the next year. When this fruit drops down all lines become *yin*, the hexagram *K'un* is formed. When the seed from this fruit sprouts, a *yang* line enters in the first place, the hexagram *Fu*/Return is formed. (*Fu* is the opposite of *Po*). Thus, in the hexagram *Po*, provision is made to obtain the seed for the next circulation of the *ch'i*.

The following lines are from the Commentary on the Decision:

> Splitting Apart means ruin. The yielding changes
>   the firm.
> Devotion and keeping still result from contemplating
>   the image. The superior man takes heed of the

> alternation of increase and decrease, fullness
> and emptiness; for it is the course of heaven.[31]

"The yielding changes the firm" describes how the lines are gradually becoming *yin*. This is essential in the practice of T'ai Chi Ch'uan because it is only when the *yang* energy has been reduced, that is, all stiffness and reliance on muscle power has been eliminated, that the exercise can be done properly.

"Devotion and keeping still" refer to the attributes of the two trigrams, *K'un* and *Ken*, which form the hexagram *Po*. They are also the attributes of the successful T'ai Chi student, thus the "superior man" here refers to the meditator or T'ai Chi player. He observes the circulation of the *ch'i*, "the course of heaven." "Increase" or spring represents the portion of the channel from the pubic region to the middle of the back. "Fullness" or summer starts at the middle of the back and goes to the back of the head (*Ch'ien*). "Decrease" or autumn drops down from the top of the head to the navel and "emptiness" or winter is the portion from the navel to the pubic region (*K'un*).

The importance of the *yin* energy is described in Chapter 48 of the *Tao Te Ching*:

> He who pursues learning will increase every day;
> He who pursues Tao will decrease every day.
> He will decrease and continue to decrease,
> Till he comes to non-action;
> By non-action everything can be done.[32]

Since T'ai Chi Ch'uan is Tao, those who practice it move in a manner soft and light as a feather, yet keep their strength within. When all the lines become *yin*, the hexagram is *K'un*/The Receptive.

K'un

K'un/The Receptive

The upper and lower trigrams are *K'un*, The Receptive, Earth.

The hexagram *K'un* means emptiness and storage. It contains six *yin* lines and is completely yielding. *K'un* represents the tenth month, November–December, the final harvest before the darkness of winter.

The trigrams of the hexagram *K'un* are also *K'un*. This hexagram represents the lower abdomen, the place where the *ch'i* will be stored until it begins the next cycle of circulation. According to the classics of T'ai Chi Ch'uan literature, "If the abdomen is relaxed and empty, the *ch'i* can penetrate to the bone. The mind remains quiet and the body at ease." This hexagram, *K'un*, is constructed of six broken lines and symbolizes the trunk of the body, which is empty and wide open. The *ch'i* can thus sink from the throat to the lower abdomen without any hindrance.

In the advanced stages of practice, the *ch'i* penetrates the bones and is stored in them, after passing through the ligaments, tendons, and joints. Many of my readers will ask: "How can the *ch'i* enter the bones, which seem to be solid?" An example drawn from practical physics may help to explain this idea, which is admittedly difficult to understand. First, it is necessary to recall a rule from the classics of T'ai Chi Ch'uan: "The mind is primary, the body is secondary. . . ." The sinking of the *ch'i* down into the abdomen composes the mind, which then directs the nerve plexus to heat the water in the abdomen so that it may become steam. It is a process similar to the way coils of an immersion heater boil water. When the moisture and blood of the body become steam, they penetrate the bones in that form. As in a steam engine, the steam can enter the "pipes" of the body, i.e., the hollow channels in the bones which contain marrow. In Taoist terminology, the practitioner must "refine the *ching* to become the *ch'i*, that is, the vitality." Also the hexagram *K'un* is characterized by softness and emptiness. It is composed of six broken lines and is explicated in the *Tao Te Ching*, Chapter 16, as follows: "Attain to the state of absolute emptiness; keep to the goal of perfect quiet." The *T'ai Chi Ch'uan Classics* says: "From being extremely soft and yielding, you will attain extreme hardness and strength." According to the hexagram *K'un*, when the six *yin* lines through process change into six *yang* lines, the hexagram becomes *Ch'ien*, which is strength and movement.

The hexagram thus no longer represents softness or emptiness. Soil becomes metal through geological changes in temperature and pressure in time. Metal becomes earth again through oxidation. This is the scientific aspect of the waxing and waning of *Ch'ien* (metal) and *K'un* (earth).

K'un represents the end of the cycle. At this point, all the *ch'i* has returned to the lower abdomen and is now quiescent. But in the quietness is the seed of movement. When all has become *yin*, the *yang* reappears. Hence, in the sixth line of the hexagram:

> Dragons fight in the meadow.
> Their blood is black and yellow.[33]

The dragons symbolize breath, energy, that is to say, the *ch'i*. Black and yellow represent *yang* and *yin*, respectively. Thus the sixth line indicates symbolically the merging of *yin* and *yang*.[34] For the moment *yin* is predominant. This phase is described by Lao Tzu in Chapter 16 of the *Tao Te Ching*:

> Things appear multitudinous and varied, but
>   eventually they all return to the common root.
> When they revert to the common root,
>   there is quiescence. The state of quiescence
>   is called the fulfilment of destiny.[35]

Thus one turn of the cycle is completed. When a *yang* line again enters at the bottom, the Hexagram 24, *Fu*/Return, is formed and the cycle begins again.

NOTES

The *I Ching* passages in this book are quoted from *The I Ching: Or Book of Changes*, translated by Richard Wilhelm, rendered into English by Cary F. Baynes (Routledge & Kegan Paul, London, 1951) and are cited by book and page number.

I. INTRODUCTION

1. Book II, pp. 348–349.

IV. THE FORMS AND THE HEXAGRAMS

1. Book III, p. 560; Book I, p. 137.
2. Book I, p. 8; Book I, p. 9; Book I, p. 9.
3. Book II, p. 280.
4. Book III, p. 636.
5. Book III, p. 474.
6. Book I, p. 134; Book I, p. 134.
7. Book I, p. 76.
8. Book I, p. 142; Book I, p. 140.
9. Book III, p. 653; Book I, pp. 201–202.
10. Book I, p. 110.
11. Book I, p. 130; Book III, p. 551.
12. Book I, p. 112.
13. Book I, p. 105.
14. Book I, p. 113; Book I, p. 114; Book I, p. 242.
15. Book I, p. 165.
16. Book I, p. 23.
17. Book I, p. 89.
18. Book I, p. 101.
19. Book I, p. 17.
20. Book I, p. 33; Book I, p. 34; Book I, p. 34.

21. Book I, p. 198.
22. Book I, p. 66; Book III, p. 465.
23. Book III, p. 695.
24. Book I, p. 213; Book I, p. 214; Book II, p. 277; Book III, p. 670.
25. Book I, p. 251.
26. Book III, p. 585.

V. T'AI CHI CH'UAN USED FOR SELF-DEFENSE

1. Book II, p. 316.

VII. THE WAXING AND WANING OF CH'IEN AND K'UN AS APPLIED TO THE PRACTICE OF T'AI CHI CH'UAN

   * T'ai Chi Ch'uan Classics says: "The feet like root of a tree, the energy moves up from the feet to the legs, directed by the waist. . . ." See T. T. Liang, *T'ai Chi Ch'uan for Health and Self-defense*, p. 19. Chuang Tze says "The breathing of the true man comes from his heels. . . ." James Legge, *The Texts of Taoism* (New York: Dover, 1962). p. 238.
1. Book III, p. 505.
2. See James Legge, *op. cit.*, p. 83.
3. Book III, p. 482.
4. Book III, p. 482.
5. Book III, p. 441.
6. Book III, p. 441.
7. Book III, p. 557.
8. Book III, p. 558.
9. Book III, p. 558.
10. Book III, p. 559.
11. Ch'u Ta-Kao, *Tao Te Ching*; see also James Legge, *op. cit.*, p. 120 and Chia-Fu Feng and Jane English, *Lao Tzu: Tao Te Ching*, Chapters 43 and 78.
12. See James Legge, *op. cit.*, p. 118.
13. Book III, p. 603.
14. Book I, p. 168.
15. See James Legge, *op. cit.*, p. 111.
16. Book I, p. 167.
17. Book I, p. 3.
18. Book I, p. 6.
19. Book I, p. 8.

20. "What is meant by 'the True man?'. . . . Being such, they could ascend the loftiest heights without fear; they could pass through water without being made wet by it; they could go into fire without being burnt;'', James Legge, *op. cit.*, p. 237.
21. Book III, p. 382. "The great man accords in his character with heaven and earth; in his light, with the sun and moon; in his consistency, with the four seasons; in the good and evil that he creates, with gods and spirits. . . ."
    † 'Chin Kang' means strong like gold. This is the attribute of the *Ch'ien* trigrams. In Sanskrit, it is the word 'vajara' which means diamond. It also refers to the four guardians of the Buddhist temples, giants of great strength.
22. See James Legge, *op. cit.*, pp. 92–3.
23. See T. T. Liang, *T'ai Chi Ch'uan for Health and Self Defense*, (New York: Random House, 1974), p. 39.
24. Book III, p. 609.
25. Book III, p. 613.
26. Book III, p. 551.
27. Book I, p. 52.
28. Book I, p. 54.
29. Book II, p. 342.
30. Book I, p. 96.
31. Book III, p. 501.
32. Ch'u Ta-Kao, *op. cit.*, p. 63.
33. Book I, p. 15.
34. In Taoist meditation, as well as in T'ai Chi Ch'uan, these two forces are joined by a chemical process. See Lu Kuang *Yü, Taoist Yoga: Alchemy and Immortality* (New York: Samuel Weiser, Inc., 1970), p. 51.
35. Cheng Lin, *The Works of Lao Tzyy* (Taipei, Taiwan: The World Book Company Ltd, 1969), p. 25.

ARKANA – NEW-AGE BOOKS FOR MIND, BODY AND SPIRIT

With over 150 titles currently in print, Arkana is the leading name in quality new-age books for mind, body and spirit. Arkana encompasses the spirituality of both East and West, ancient and new, in fiction and non-fiction. A vast range of interests is covered, including Psychology and Transformation, Health, Science and Mysticism, Women's Spirituality and Astrology.

If you would like a catalogue of Arkana books, please write to:

Arkana Marketing Department
Penguin Books Ltd
27 Wright's Lane
London W8 5TZ

ARKANA - NEW-AGE BOOKS FOR MIND, BODY AND SPIRIT

A selection of titles already published or in preparation

Neal's Yard Natural Remedies Susan Curtis, Romy Fraser and Irene Kohler

Natural remedies for common ailments from the pioneering Neal's Yard Apothecary Shop. An invaluable resource for everyone wishing to take responsibility for their own health, enabling you to make your own choice from homeopathy, aromatherapy and herbalism.

The Arkana Dictionary of New Perspectives Stuart Holroyd

Clear, comprehensive and compact, this iconoclastic reference guide brings together the orthodox and the highly unorthodox, doing full justice to *every* facet of contemporary thought – psychology and parapsychology, culture and counter-culture, science and so-called pseudo-science.

The Absent Father: Crisis and Creativity Alix Pirani

Freud used Oedipus to explain human nature; but Alix Pirani believes that the myth of Danae and Perseus has most to teach an age which offers 'new responsibilities for women and challenging questions for men' – a myth which can help us face the darker side of our personalities and break the patterns inherited from our parents.

Woman Awake: A Celebration of Women's Wisdom Christina Feldman

In this inspiring book, Christina Feldman suggests that it *is* possible to break out of those negative patterns instilled into us by our social conditioning as women: confirmity, passivity and surrender of self. Through a growing awareness of the dignity of all life and its connection with us, we can regain our sense of power and worth.

Water and Sexuality Michel Odent

Taking as his starting point his world-famous work on underwater childbirth at Pithiviers, Michel Odent considers the meaning and importance of water as a symbol: in the past – expressed through myths and legends – and today, from an advertisers' tool to a metaphor for aspects of the psyche. Dr Odent also boldly suggests that the human species may have had an aquatic past.

ARKANA – NEW-AGE BOOKS FOR MIND, BODY AND SPIRIT

A selection of titles already published or in preparation

Head Off Stress: Beyond the Bottom Line D. E. Harding

Learning to head off stress takes no time at all and is impossible to forget – all it requires is that we dare take a fresh look at ourselves. This infallible and revolutionary guide from the author of *On Having No Head* – whose work C. S. Lewis described as 'highest genius' – shows how.

Shiatzu: Japanese Finger Pressure for Energy, Sexual Vitality and Relief from Tension and Pain
Yukiko Irwin with James Wagenvoord

The product of 4000 years of Oriental medicine and philosophy, Shiatzu is a Japanese variant of the Chinese practice of acupuncture. Fingers, thumbs and palms are applied to the 657 pressure points that the Chinese penetrate with gold and silver needles, aiming to maintain health, increase vitality and promote well-being.

The Magus of Strovolos: The Extraordinary World of a Spiritual Healer Kyriacos C. Markides

This vivid account introduces us to the rich and intricate world of Daskalos, the Magus of Strovolos – a true healer who draws upon a seemingly limitless mixture of esoteric teachings, psychology, reincarnation, demonology, cosmology and mysticism, from both East and West.

'This is a really marvellous book . . . one of the most extraordinary accounts of a "magical" personality since Ouspensky's account of Gurdjieff' – Colin Wilson

Meetings With Remarkable Men G. I. Gurdjieff

All that we know of the early life of Gurdjieff – one of the great spiritual masters of this century – is contained within these colourful and profound tales of adventure. The men who influenced his formative years had no claim to fame in the conventional sense; what made them remarkable was the consuming desire they all shared to understand the deepest mysteries of life.

ARKANA – NEW-AGE BOOKS FOR MIND, BODY AND SPIRIT

A selection of titles already published or in preparation

The TM Technique Peter Russell

Through a process precisely opposite to that by which the body accumulates stress and tension, transcendental meditation works to produce a state of profound rest, with positive benefits for health, clarity of mind, creativity and personal stability. Peter Russell's book has become the key work for everyone requiring a complete mastery of TM.

The Development of the Personality: Seminars in Psychological Astrology Volume I Liz Greene and Howard Sasportas

Taking as a starting point their groundbreaking work on the cross-fertilization between astrology and psychology, Liz Greene and Howard Sasportas show how depth psychology works with the natal chart to illuminate the experiences and problems all of us encounter throughout the development of our individual identity, from childhood onwards.

Homage to the Sun: The Wisdom of the Magus of Strovolos Kyriacos C. Markides

Homage to the Sun continues the adventure into the mysterious and extraordinary world of the spiritual teacher and healer Daskalos, the 'Magus of Strovolos'. The logical foundations of Daskalos' world of other dimensions are revealed to us – invisible masters, past-life memories and guardian angels, all explained by the Magus with great lucidity and scientific precision.

The Year I: Global Process Work Arnold Mindell

As we approach the end of the 20th century, we are on the verge of planetary extinction. Solving the planet's problems is literally a matter of life and death. Arnold Mindell shows how his famous and groundbreaking process-orientated psychology can be extended so that our own sense of global awareness can be developed and we – the whole community of earth's inhabitants – can comprehend the problems and work together towards solving them.

ARKANA – NEW-AGE BOOKS FOR MIND, BODY AND SPIRIT

A selection of titles already published or in preparation

Being Intimate: A Guide to Successful Relationships
John and Kris Amodeo

This invaluable guide aims to enrich one of the most important – yet often problematic – aspects of our lives: intimate relationships and friendships.

'A clear and practical guide to the realization and communication of authentic feelings, and thus an excellent pathway towards lasting intimacy and love' – George Leonard

The Brain Book Peter Russell

The essential handbook for brain users.

'A fascinating book – for everyone who is able to appreciate the human brain, which, as Russell says, is the most complex and most powerful information processor known to man. It is especially relevant for those who are called upon to read a great deal when time is limited, or who attend lectures or seminars and need to take notes' – *Nursing Times*

The Act of Creation Arthur Koestler

This second book in Koestler's classic trio of works on the human mind (which opened with *The Sleepwalkers* and concludes with *The Ghost in the Machine*) advances the theory that all creative activities – the conscious and unconscious processes underlying artistic originality, scientific discovery and comic inspiration – share a basic pattern, which Koestler expounds and explores with all his usual clarity and brilliance.

A Psychology With a Soul: Psychosynthesis in Evolutionary Context Jean Hardy

Psychosynthesis was developed between 1910 and the 1950s by Roberto Assagioli – an Italian psychiatrist who, like Jung, diverged from Freud in search of a more spiritually based understanding of human nature. Jean Hardy's account of this comprehensive approach to self-realization will be of great value to everyone concerned with personal integration and spiritual growth.

ARKANA – NEW-AGE BOOKS FOR MIND, BODY AND SPIRIT

A selection of titles already published or in preparation

The Networking Book: People Connecting with People
Jessica Lipnack and Jeffrey Stamps

Networking – forming human connections to link ideas and resources – is the natural form of organization for an era based on information technology. Principally concerned with those networks whose goal is a peaceful yet dynamic future for the world, *The Networking Book* – written by two world-famous experts – profiles hundreds of such organizations worldwide, operating at every level from global tele-communications to word of mouth.

Chinese Massage Therapy: A Handbook of Therapeutic Massage Compiled at the Anhui Medical School Hospital, China
Translated by Hor Ming Lee and Gregory Whincup

There is a growing movement among medical practitioners in China today to mine the treasures of traditional Chinese medicine – acupuncture, herbal medicine and massage therapy. Directly trans-lated from a manual in use in Chinese hospitals, *Chinese Massage Therapy* offers a fresh understanding of this time-tested medical alternative.

Dialogues with Scientists and Sages: The Search for Unity
Renée Weber

In their own words, contemporary scientists and mystics – from the Dalai Lama to Stephen Hawking – share with us their richly diverse views on space, time, matter, energy, life, consciousness, creation and our place in the scheme of things. Through the immediacy of verbatim dialogue, we encounter scientists who endorse mysticism, and those who oppose it; mystics who dismiss science, and those who embrace it.

Zen and the Art of Calligraphy
Omōri Sōgen and Terayama Katsujo

Exploring every element of the relationship between Zen thought and the artistic expression of calligraphy, two long-time practitioners of Zen, calligraphy and swordsmanship show how Zen training provides a proper balance of body and mind, enabling the calligrapher to write more profoundly, freed from distraction or hesitation.

ARKANA – NEW-AGE BOOKS FOR MIND, BODY AND SPIRIT

A selection of titles already published or in preparation

The Ghost in the Machine Arthur Koestler

Koestler's classic work – which can be read alone or as the conclusion of his trilogy on the human mind – is concerned not with human creativity but with human pathology.

'He has seldom been as impressive, as scientifically far-ranging, as lively-minded or as alarming as on the present occasion' – John Raymond in the *Financial Times*

T'ai Chi Ch'uan and Meditation Da Liu

Today T'ai Chi Ch'uan is known primarily as a martial art – but it was originally developed as a complement to meditation. Both disciplines involve alignment of the self with the Tao, the ultimate reality of the universe. Da Liu shows how to combine T'ai Chi Ch'uan and meditation, balancing the physical and spiritual aspects to attain good health and harmony with the universe.

Return of the Goddess Edward C. Whitmont

Amidst social upheaval and the questioning of traditional gender roles, a new myth is arising: the myth of the ancient Goddess who once ruled earth and heaven before the advent of patriarchy and patriachal religion. Here one of the world's leading Jungian analysts argues that our society, long dominated by male concepts of power and aggression, is today experiencing a resurgence of the feminine.

The Strange Life of Ivan Osokin P. D. Ouspensky

If you had the chance to live your life again, what would you do with it? Ouspensky's novel, set in Moscow, on a country estate and in Paris, tells what happens to Ivan Ososkin when he is sent back twelve years to his stormy schooldays, early manhood and early loves. First published in 1947, the *Manchester Guardian* praised it as 'a brilliant fantasy . . . written to illustrate the theme that we do not live life but that life lives us'.